Praise

"For a topic area that is full of strong opinions and dogma, *Feed the Baby* is a refreshingly inclusive, nonjudgmental companion ready to be by your side, cheering you on on your unique feeding journey."

—Katherine Goldstein, journalist and creator of *The Double Shift*

"This is the kind of book that [we] have dreamed of writing and is the perfect step-by-step guide to feeding your baby, complete with illustrations and videos. Victoria Facelli is an internationally board-certified lactation consultant, but not the kind that hates formula. She wrote this book to cut through a lot of the misinformation that parents are faced with, as a resource to empower parents to feed their babies in whatever way works for them!"

—Heather ONeal, CNM, IBCLC, and
Maureen Farrell, CLC, DEM, hosts of the *Milk Minute Podcast*

"*Feed the Baby* is a must-read for new parents. It provides a wealth of information based on research and experience from the author . . . [and] takes a nonjudgmental approach to guide parents through the ever-changing first several years of feeding an infant and early toddler. . . . Even better, this book is not just for parents. It has something for everyone who makes up the village that helps nurture a newborn. *Feed the Baby* has already helped me provide better guidance to new parents in my practice and is an easy recommendation."

—Michael DiBartola, MD, pediatrician, Columbus OH

FEED THE BABY

FEED THE BABY.

An Inclusive Guide to Nursing, Bottle-Feeding & Everything in Between

Victoria Facelli, IBCLC

FOREWORD BY
Shruti Nagaraj, MD, MPH

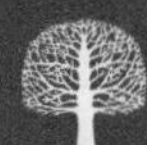

Countryman Press

An Imprint of W. W. Norton & Company
Celebrating a Century of Independent Publishing

Feed the Baby is a work of nonfiction. Some potentially identifying characteristics, including names, dialogue, and visual depictions, have been changed.

Printed in the United States of America
First published as a Countryman Press paperback 2025

For information about permission to reproduce selections from this book, write to Permissions, Countryman Press, 500 Fifth Avenue, New York, NY 10110

For information about special discounts for bulk purchases, please contact W. W. Norton Special Sales at specialsales@wwnorton.com or 800-233-4830

Manufacturing by Lake Book Manufacturing
Book design by Allison Chi

Countryman Press
www.countrymanpress.com

An imprint of W. W. Norton & Company, Inc.
500 Fifth Avenue, New York, NY 10110
www.wwnorton.com

ISBN 978-1-68268-966-0 pbk.

10 9 8 7 6 5 4 3 2 1

For my mom, Ana Maria,
who taught me to be a force.

CONTENTS

SECTION FOUR.
Help for When It's Not Working

FOREWORD

SHRUTI NAGARAJ, MD, MPH

On the third day in the hospital after I gave birth to my child I was told by my nurse, "Well, of course breastfeeding is best . . . and after that comes breast milk that you can get from a family member or a friend and then. . . . *way* lower [dropping her hand and motioning low to the ground] comes formula."

I've been in pediatrics for ten years, but in that moment, I was just a new mom. I attended University of North Carolina-Chapel Hill for undergrad, a master's in public health, and medical school, followed by a residency at University of California, Los Angeles. I've worked everywhere, from community hospitals, community clinics, and private practice to the mountains of Honduras. My background in public health helps me think critically about the whole picture when I see patients. I care for babies daily and answer their family's questions about everything from nipple confusion to hiccups. I comfort families when they are in tears and worried about their baby's weight gain.

Yet despite the professional expertise, knowledge, and reassurance I give parents daily, this comment caused me to start spiraling: What if *I* can't breastfeed? How do I rationalize giving my baby something that makes someone point SO low to the ground when talking about it? Do I know anyone who has extra milk? Am I in a milk-sharing Facebook group? Am I okay with milk sharing? Do I even still have an active Facebook account? Am I setting my child up for failure . . . on her third day of life?!

In that moment, I was seeing things as a new parent, not as a doctor, and I felt the deep sense of anxiety many of my patients must feel when figuring out how to feed a baby. For most of us, it is *not* a linear path, and treating it as a binary issue (breast milk versus formula) fails to recognize how complicated this experience is. Comments like "breastfeeding is best" reinforce the judgment and shame around a choice to even use formula.

That's where this book comes in. Patients ask me daily for book recommendations about every baby topic imaginable. This is one I will hand them when they ask about feeding their baby.

This book is what I wish I'd had on my bedstand to read during the middle-of-the-night feeds, instead of searching for answers on social media. *Feed the Baby* shares the experiences of other families and reassures us that we are not alone in feeling confused by it all. Victoria Facelli is a master of simplifying what may seem overwhelming. She provides solid data sprinkled with relatable stories. She helps us to see what feeding a baby really looks like. As a clinician, I know that my patients want to be educated without being forced in a direction. To know they won't be judged for however they decide to do things. Here is the updated guidance that is applicable to the world we live in today.

You may think becoming a mother after being a pediatrician means that I know what I'm doing. You'd be wrong. But I do know these things for certain:

- Feeding your baby is one of the best (and worst) experiences a parent has—it's relentless, it's necessary, and can be wonderful.
- A parent's mental health is equally important to, if not more important than, breastfeeding.
- No one can tell you exactly how to feed your baby.
- You don't need anyone's permission to change your mind about any part of this.
- I would have stopped breastfeeding very early if it weren't for my partner and my pediatrician (yes, pediatricians' kids have pediatricians too). It's necessary to rely on things outside of yourself to help you through this process.

If you're like me and sometimes skip to the end hoping for a punchy digest, here goes: The best way to feed a baby is the way that works for you. Give yourself time to figure it out. Go into the process armed with reliable information, few expectations, and a very low tolerance for judgement. And as always, feed the baby.

INTRODUCTION

This is a book about feeding babies. Nothing more, nothing less.

It's easy in the early days of parenthood to confuse feeding with parenting. It is how you will spend most of your time in the beginning. It is, of course, not parenting. It is certainly not what defines parenting. That being said, it's not uncommon for parents whose feeding plan comes easily to feel like a success, while those who struggle feel like they are a failure. This—combined with a narrative about what's "best" to do—can be deeply demoralizing during what is already a fragile time.

You won't find any words like "best" or "success" here. I'll assume that just like me, you are getting through the day, trying to make sure that at the end of it, the baby is alive and no one lost their job or their mind. My hope is that you navigate feeding your baby with knowledge, a little humility, and a laugh or two. I hope to get you through this first challenge of parenting and on to the part where the child embarrasses you at restaurants, which is a much larger part of being a parent.

I am not here to explain why you should feed your baby a certain way. There are far more ways than one to feed a baby. Formula feeding, nursing, pumping, bottle feeding, and giving a baby donor milk are all common and healthy options. It is unhelpful to classify one form of feeding as a success and condemn the others as failures. Instead of dogma, I am offering you tools. In this book you will learn the science of how and why babies eat the way they do and how humans make milk the way we do. This knowledge will help you make choices and changes as you go. I want you to be a uniquely qualified expert on your body, your baby, and your life. This expertise will allow you to wield the available baby-feeding tools to serve your family, in your way, on your terms. I hope these tools empower your family to make sustainable choices for your babies and yourselves. Babies are hard, and wonderful. Feeding can be equally hard and equally wonderful. I hope that feeding your baby starts off a life of enjoying food together and sharing of yourself and your culture.

How to read this book: You, dear reader, fall into one of two categories: you are either expecting a baby in your life, or you already have one. The first section of this book is jam-packed with info about how to prep for your baby. The rest follows a rough chronology of newborn, infant, and toddler development. This is to make each section easy to refer back to when you need help quickly, and also because you may experience that specific situation sooner or later (or not at all) during your baby's first year, or you may not experience it just the once (yep, feeding can be unpredictable). At the end of the book you'll find some answers to your panicked questions. If it's 3 a.m. and you are up with worry that your kid won't take a bottle at daycare next week, or the baby won't latch, that section will quickly give you what you need, or refer you back to the right place, so you can get back to sleep.

You can read this book cover to cover, or section to section as you go. If your baby is not yet earthside, I recommend reading through at least week two for a good survey of your options and what to expect during the most hectic part of newbornhood. If you already have a baby in your arms, jump right to the sections you need and know that much of the background info is right there for you to refer back to. You'll notice that the timeline fluctuates. This reflects the experience of feeding babies: it gets easier as you go, so hang in there, but there are hard bits that are pretty common to most parents.

In the words of brilliant doctor of breastfeeding medicine and OB-GYN Alison Stuebe, "I believe there is far more common ground than controversy—and that it is from this common ground that we will build a society that truly supports families."

This book is for my generation of parents, a group I have come to know well. We are working hard to parent and co-parent in efficient and egalitarian ways. We are trying to know absolutely everything we can about everything we do. We read reviews and survey our friends. We make plans and expect to have all of the information to make informed choices.

> **"Rather than squabble about the extent to which breastfeeding impacts biomedical outcomes, we should fight for the rights of mothers to decide how care for their children and enable them to do so, thereby improving health and well-being across two generations."**
>
> **—DR. ALISON STUEBE**

This book is for all of us. It is not only for a white lady with bangs gazing into her baby's eyes while she breastfeeds, though she is welcome to join us. As a queer, autistic Latina woman with a disabled child, I just don't see myself in her, and I found that most of my clients didn't either. Feeding babies is more complicated than that image, and so are our identities and relationships to parenting. It is for dads, trans parents, Black and brown parents, foster parents, Indigenous parents, disabled parents, grandparents, and anyone else who is feeding a baby. It's for the women who look just like the breastfeeding poster-mom, but sure as hell don't feel like her. You'll find some of their stories woven into individual chapters. I hope you see yourself in them and love them for their differences too. If a section of this book doesn't fit your specific situation, lifestyle, or identity, I invite readers to skip over it or cross it out. It'll be there if the situation changes.

I know a little something about situations changing.

I am the lactation consultant who couldn't feed her kid.

That's a bit of an exaggeration, but this felt true to me once. I was a lactation consultant long before I was a mother. I was a postpartum doula before that, and a nanny before that. I had probably assisted in feeding over a hundred babies in the decade before I made and met my own. My daughter is bright, hilarious, beautiful, and driven as hell. She was also born not breathing, and as a result has cerebral palsy (a motor disability), and that impacts how she eats. No amount of training, experience, or will power on my end was going to change that.

This kind of birth event is rare, but as I had learned in the previous decade, feeding challenges are not. Despite spending my days with people crying over every possible feeding complication, I expected my experience to be different. I had the know-how to do it right. I knew how to prevent early engorgement, how to hand-express colostrum, I had AFFIRMATIONS, for goodness' sake. I was prepared. I could latch a piranha on a watermelon, I'm that good at my job.

There I was with two doulas, a midwife, an OB-GYN, and an awesome partner at my side, and I still had no control of where I ended up. Which for me, was the NICU and unable to feed my baby. My head was swimming with hormones and confusion as my daughter's neonatologist discussed feeding tubes and outcomes. I just stared at the total parental nutrition (TPN)—weird and miraculous complete nutrition that looks like flubber, a personalized blend of water, energy, fat, vitamins, and minerals that is made to go directly into the veins, rather than being digested. It is a miracle of science and one that I was blissfully unaware of until that moment. It was injected into my daughter's bloodstream via her heart: thanks, science. I turned to my sister, who had boarded a plane hours after my daughter was born and said, "I am supposed to be a feeding expert, and I can't feed her."

Of course, I did feed her. I fed her via a feeding tube, and then via bottles. I fed her expressed breast milk for nine months and formula after that. I nursed her at the breast successfully exactly once. It was a tiny miracle that I will hold onto forever. It wasn't a miracle because it was breastfeeding. It was a miracle because it was one tiny slice of the imagined reality I thought I would get.

I worked very hard on breastfeeding with some of the most amazing bodyworkers, speech therapists, doctors, and lactation consultants I know.

We revised her tongue-tie, used a supplementary nursing system, tried shields, tried everything. She was genuinely only able to drink from the bottle. Finally, I let breastfeeding go. In the spirit of doing everything I could for her health, I pumped like every good NICU parent is told to. I, the formula-positive, choice-focused lactation consultant, forgot everything I believed about family well-being and risk/benefits. I was so focused on doing anything I could for her health that I did what I had never imagined I would do and exclusively pumped for nine months. I pumped through a suicidal mood disorder, through a colonoscopy, through a gruelling schedule of my kid's appointments. I pumped and pumped and pumped until I was so sick from mastitis and colitis from treating the mastitis that I was in excruciating pain and a diaper due to a torn rectum from her birth. Then, I let the pumping go, too.

Letting go was the hardest thing I've ever done, and I am so proud. I am also proud that I tried. I am proud that I pumped for so long. I am proud that I survived PTSD, a postpartum mood disorder with suicidal thoughts, and all my grief to become a badass queer Latina mom with a badass family and a badass disabled kid.

She and I aren't in the other books on infant feeding and baby care. Disabled kids, disabled parents, queer parents, parents making really complicated choices in a really complicated world: We aren't in there. So I wrote this book for us.

I am writing this book so that you can become the parent you are meant to be, too. Proud of achieving what you set out to do, but equally proud of letting things go when they aren't working. I encourage changing your mind and changing course. I hope you choose your mental health and joy over any ideas you have about succeeding. I hope this book helps you thrive, just like my family did.

Dear partners, dads and non-gestational parents, support people, this is your feeding journey, too. Some of you may plan to be the primary stay-at-home parent, some of you may only get a few days' leave. This is still your feeding experience, too. You should plan to be involved in helping with feedings and navigating feeding choices.

While all of the content in this book is going to help you support your family, if you don't have time to read everything, here is where to start:

- Bottle-feeding (page 35)
- Baby cues (page 189)
- Milk processing and storage (page 236)
- Supporting nursing positioning (page 107)

A NOTE ON REPRESENTATION

This book is not only for women, and certainly not for one kind of woman. Many cisgender dads bottle feed babies, and parents of all genders may use their bodies to feed babies. I will use the word *breast* throughout the book as a clinical term and *chest* as an umbrella term, but I invite the reader to cross it out and use the word they prefer. I primarily use the word *nursing* to refer to feeding a baby at the chest. There are many ways that people define breastfeeding, human milk–feeding and bottle feeding. I strive to use as inclusive and specific language as I can without getting too confusing.

I would also like to take a moment to acknowledge the systemic oppression of Black people in infant mortality and infant feeding. I am not Black and cannot fully understand the way that the history of enslaved wet-nursing and inadequate healthcare for Black families is sewn into Black parenting. While I include representation of Black bodies and Black voices, the work to be done in this area is immense, and I will continue to seek out anti-racist approaches to healthcare and Black-led initiatives around feeding.

This book was written on the unceded territory of several Native nations, including Tutelo- and Saponi-speaking peoples. For more resources on Native breast- and chestfeeding, I direct you to the work of the Indigenous Milk Medicine Collective, who can speak directly to Native infant-feeding experiences and direct you to Native feeding resources and support.

QR codes. In this book you will see QR codes that will take you to video content related to that section. These pertain to feeding techniques that are best shown as well as explained. This QR code will take you to a list of all the QR codes in the book, or you can find them as you go.

SECTION ONE

YOUR FEEDING JOURNEY.

CHAPTER 1

GETTING STARTED

Babies begin swallowing in utero at about fifteen weeks of pregnancy. This is also the time when those of us overachiever, type A, prep parents start devouring books and blogs and researching strollers. If I'm being honest: I started decades before my baby was twelve weeks along. I became interested in this field when, as a nanny, I would read parenting books at nap time. I became the world's foremost childless expert on picky eaters, sleeping babies, and car seats: as only someone who doesn't have actual children can be. This led to being a postpartum doula, and as I watched completely prepared parents struggle with feeding, I set out to learn more and eventually became an actual expert on the subject. I became what is known as an international board certified lactation consultant (IBCLC)—meaning I did hundreds of hours of time in lectures and working with parents and took a very, very long exam on the subject. I adore parents who like to prepare. I loved teaching feeding classes to expecting parents. I loved helping adoptive parents put all that waiting to good use. What I learned both in my work and in my life was that expectant parents develop grandiose ideas about how to feed their babies. Ideally, they get set up with the supplies and supports they will need in early parenthood. However, some aspects of feeding your baby can be planned, and some can't. Some are in your control; a lot aren't. The goal of this book is for you to find your own right path and make sure you feel supported along the way.

Babies get fed two main ways: at the breast/chest and with a bottle.

Bottle-fed babies drink formula or pumped milk. Sounds simple enough, right? Some people have a clear plan to exclusively formula feed; many people do some combination of nursing, pumping, and formula feeding at some point in their babies' early years. Nursing is at its base a closed-loop system, and there can be a great ease in that. Your body makes enough food for your baby, they drink it right from the tap, and tada! But for most of us—not getting enough leave or wanting to work, needing sleep or time to care for ourselves, encountering medical roadblocks or a lack of desire to feed that way—it is almost never that simple.

This time before your baby is born is the time to set intentions and gather enough information to change course temporarily, or long term, as needed. I often think of formula feeding like walking. It's fairly straightforward for most people, but remains constant in the amount of effort. Nursing is like driving. It's really intense and nerve-racking while you get the hang of it, but once you have it down, you rarely even have to think about it. Meanwhile, pumping is like cross-country skiing. It's straightforward, but always a whole lot of effort. Since most families will use a combination of tools, first let's understand the methods (look under the hood, if you will) and how they interact with each other.

Most people have a lot of ideas about how they want to feed their baby; that's great. Some people come with a lot of unknowns, or a history related to feeding past babies, or chest surgery, or of family dynamics around feeding. Wherever you are coming from, it's good to take stock of what you are bringing with you. I recommend taking some time to think about, journal about, and discuss these ideas with your primary support person/co-parent. Knowing where you are coming from will help you understand where you are going.

It is important to sit with the benefits of each kind of feeding and to think about why they are important to you. This not only centers you strongly in your choices but will help you shift plans if need be. For each type of feeding, I'll work through the pros and cons, what you'll need and how to get set up. Later in the book, I'll explain the specifics involved in each choice.

Here are some things for you to think about:

- If equal bonding with both parents is important to you, you may want to discuss using bottles and what you want to put in these bottles. Or if you both have the ability and desire to lactate, you can discuss sharing nursing.
- If breast milk feeding is extremely important to you, then nursing, pumped milk, and donor milk are going to be your preferred options.
- If being able to devote yourself fully back to your work life is important to you, you may choose to nurse when you are home and do bottles when you return to work. Or exclusively formula feed.

Parents often blame themselves when things don't go to plan. So, let's try to make plans that set you up for success but also acknowledge the things that are out of (or mostly out of) our control.

What's in Your Control

- Where you give birth (most of the time)
- Finding a support network
- Understanding your personal anatomy
- Acquiring pumps, bottles, formula

What's Not in Your Control

- Your baby's personality, health or anatomy
- Your anatomy
- How your baby is born
- Feeding choices if you are fostering a baby

Other Things to Consider

- Your health matters, too

ՊՊՊՊ

There is a dangerous little phrase that drifts through our society: "Healthy parent, healthy baby." *What kind of birth do you want? I don't care, as long as we are both healthy. The baby is here! Both mom and baby are healthy.* It's innocuous enough, because what it means is that both birthing person and baby navigated the complex waters of birth safely. This phrase, however, negates those of us who aren't "healthy" or "happy." What we need in this time is more support, not an exclusion that makes us feel like failures. For me, my episiotomy recovery fell sacrifice to pumping. So did my mental health. I want to say right here at the beginning of the book that you are allowed to and should prioritize your health when making feeding choices for your family—specifically, whether you use breast milk or formula, and how you'll feed that breast milk or formula to your baby. While most drugs are compatible with nursing, it is wise to choose a drug you need over breast-milk feeding. It is okay to choose sleep for well-being, mental health, or physical recovery over exclusivity or one kind of feeding. It is good to ask for help, and it is a sign of a good parent to change your mind about things to meet changing needs.

As for what it really feels like to go from growing a baby with your body to feeding it that way: it's a lot. You may have experienced in pregnancy, whether you were carrying or not, that people view your body as public. Advice on what to eat or do abounds, from family and strangers alike. Feel free to ignore all of this advice. The "I formula fed, and my kids turned out fine" is just as useless as the "You really must breastfeed; it's so much healthier." None of these people are you or your baby, and so they lack a lot of the key information about what you need.

You will also experience some very significant body changes as your body goes from growing a human to feeding one. Oh, and sagginess-wise, the deed is done. It is pregnancy that changes breast length, not nursing. (This is one of my all-time favorite studies, because I like to imagine people coming in over time to have their chest length measured.) As a pregnant parent, your body will go through some kind of a milk transition, regardless of whether you are planning to nurse, though I can give you tools to make this more comfortable in either case. Birth recovery pain is to be expected and can impact feeding and mood. Most babies and parents aren't amazing at nursing right out of the gate, so anticipate experiencing some pain and needing a little help.

Speaking of help, now is a good time to take stock of who is on your team.

- Who do you imagine helping you in these early days?
- Does your birth place have best practices to support your feeding plan? Have you discussed it with your team to make sure they respect your wishes?
- Are you and your partner on the same page about how you want to feed your baby?
- Are any caregivers coming to help out after your baby is born? It's a good idea to fill them in on the plans and how they can best support you.

If this isn't your first rodeo, this is also a good moment to assess what happened last time. If you are reading this book before the arrival of your second, third, fourth, *n*th kid, I'm guessing last time there were some things that you would like to go more smoothly this time. You may not have control over all the variables (introducing a whole new person—or people, in the case of multiples—will bring its own issues). When you are reconstructing what happened last time, try to find a reliable narrator, a good friend whom you talked to a lot then, a lactation consultant or doula you worked with, a partner, or your mom. Hopefully they can help you figure out what happened last time and if any challenges were the result of:

You

- Breast anatomy
- Thyroid function
- Hemorrhage
- Chest anatomy

Your baby

- Tongue-tie
- Positional symmetry
- Disability

Your circumstances

- Birth recovery
- Lack of support
- Work schedule
- Natural disaster

Once you parse out a bit more of what happened last time, you can begin to understand what is and isn't in your control; what is likely to be different this time and what isn't.

Finally, there are A LOT of products related to feeding babies. As I work through the different types of feeding, I'll list both what you need and what you might like to have for each type of feeding, so that you'll be prepared whatever your initial plan was. I love strollers and car seats. I can talk about the pros and cons of every single one for actual days. My happy place is a screened porch, a martini, and a baby expo being livestreamed on social media. You may be like me and want All. The. Things. Or you just want what is absolutely essential. Specific suggestions will come in the relevant feeding sections, and I'll give my ratings of how necessary each item is.

Ready?

Of course not. You can never be truly ready to welcome a baby into your family, but you'll do great, I promise. Sit with this information for a bit. Examine the biases and values you are bringing with you. Talk to your family and co-parents about what is important and how you can work together. Talk through any disagreements now.

I have a lot of tools in this book, but as for advice, the best I have is to rest when you can and be ready to change with the circumstances.

CHAPTER 2

NURSING, BOTTLE FEEDING, AND EVERYTHING IN BETWEEN

To start with, there are a few must-have items regardless of how you choose to feed your baby:

Cloths. Maybe the least glamorous and most necessary baby item is a whole lot of cloths: wash cloths, towels, burps cloths, trifold cloth diapers, or receiving blankets. Babies are drippy and dribbly—so are postpartum chests. The wiping up of drips, spills, spit-up, and dribbles is constant. Cloths can also do double duty helping you get set up to comfortably feed a baby, whether by chest or bottle.

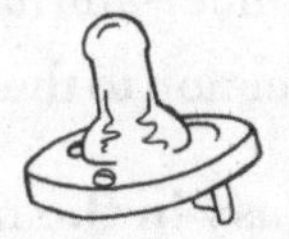

Pacifiers. I recommend pacifiers that have a straight tip for developing a correct suck (page 202). Babies need to suck a lot, so having pacifiers around can be a big help for most. A parent's clean finger will also work just fine. I don't recommend using pacifiers before two weeks, as they can hide feeding cues, but from there on out, go for it. The big exception here is premature babies. They need to suck for brain development and will be given pacifiers in the NICU.

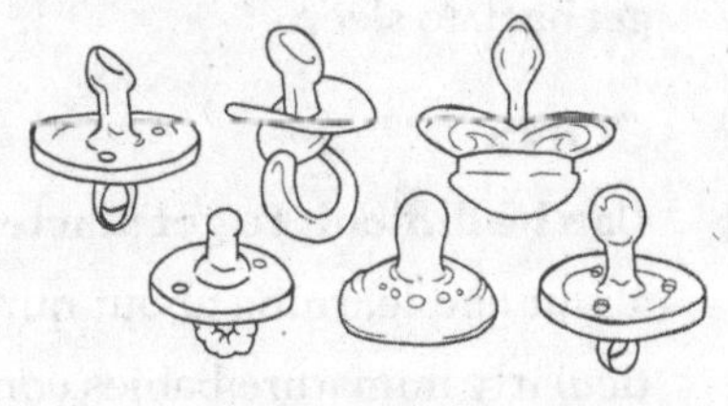

A safe place to set your baby down. This can be a bassinet, a firm bed with the comforters pulled back, a crib, or a sturdy box a la a Scandinavian baby box. But you definitely need a safe place to set your baby down when you are exhausted or frustrated.

NURSING

Biologically, nursing is a baseline. A lot of people start here and see where it goes. There is a perception that because nursing is "natural" it is easy to do. That's false. For people who are able to get in a groove, it can be awesome and very easy once they get going.

PROS

As mammals, we are mostly designed for it. There are lots of neat little aspects of development and body feeding that we may never know the full scope of. Some researchers consider it the healthiest option. Health is complicated, but the population-wide benefits of nursing babies is undeniable.

Portable all-the-time food. Carrying perpetual food with you can make things like travel and outings simpler, and can help in times of evacuation or disaster.

Bonding. A lot of parents (though, and I cannot stress this enough, not all) really like nursing and find it helps them bond. Some parents find it really gender-affirming; some nongenetic parents really like this biological connection to their babies.

Easy in the middle of the night. If you don't have help overnight and nursing is going well, nursing is the least effortful way to feed a baby and get back to sleep.

CONS

Can be difficult to get started. Most of us don't spend much time talking about and learning about nursing before we have kids, and we have particularly immature babies compared to other mammals. That means that nursing is HARD. With the right support, it's possible and, for a lot of parents, worth it. Get to know your body (see "Nursing," page 89) if nursing is part of your ideal feeding plan.

Closed-loop system is delicate. Milk production is a delicate supply-and-demand system, especially in the first six weeks. That means that using some bottles or pumping too much during this time can result in too little or too much milk, which is hard to course correct.

Some people just don't make milk, and some babies just can't nurse. My baby couldn't nurse. My best friend didn't make milk. Even the most nursing-focused and best-resourced parents can't make it work sometimes, and that's okay. Bodies are different and fallible, and it's ableist and unhelpful to think otherwise.

WHAT YOU'LL NEED

First, remember: It's the 2020s. Almost anything can be brought to you within a few hours at a push of a button, so there is no need to have everything right now. For instance, if you plan to nurse but are leaving the door open to formula feeding, you can change course easily by ordering those items as you need them or buying them at a store. I love when people change their mind, and that doesn't mean you need to have all of the things for every circumstance before your baby arrives.

Must have

Pillows and towels. Early on, it can take a lot of pillows to get a floppy newborn in the right position to latch correctly. A nursing pillow should have a firm, flat surface, so you can use firm bed pillows or towels if you can't or don't want to buy anything new.

Some pillows I recommend are:

- My Brest Friend travel nursing pillow—This is great for people with relatively little storage who plan to use it again for other babies.
- Frida Mom nursing pillow—Simple and great.
- The Nesting Pillow—A giant sack of barley that doubles as a weighted blanket.

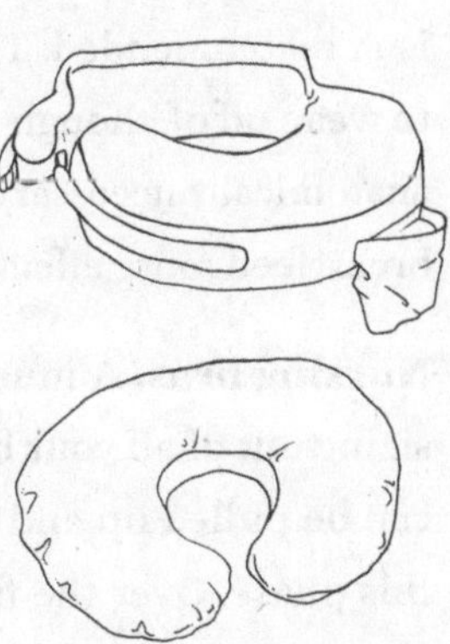

There are many others on the market, but the main thing you are looking for is that it lies flush to your body and is firm and flat. U-shaped pillows that dip in middle create a baby-shaped cavern that is very frustrating for feeding.

For multiples:

- My Brest Friend twin pillow—Otherwise known as the world's largest fanny pack/the thing that could have saved Jack on the *Titanic*.

Nipple cream. Nipple healing in the early days when you are getting the hang of things takes milk and moisture. After you nurse, I recommend expressing a little milk and following that up with some kind of moisturizer/"goop." Goop needs to be baby safe, but there is no evidence that supports one goop over another. You can buy one of the million preformulated ones or use Vaseline or coconut oil. Goop can also be used when pumping to lubricate flanges (the parts of the pump that make contact with your body), covered on page 156.

Nipple shields. These are a must-have for some bodies. This is like a little silicon hat that goes over the nipple for breastfeeding. It is very frustratingly misnamed, and I invite you to think of it as a nipple extender, as shields are excellent for parents who have flat or inverted nipples (see page 94), to shape their nipple so that it is easier for a baby to latch onto. They are not, however, a pain shield and are often misused this way. Using them as a shield will often cause tissue damage or hide other feeding issues, so it isn't recommended. They are also a little habit-forming and can take time to wean off of, though there is no need to wean off of using them if they are anatomically necessary for you. They have also been shown to help preemies breastfeed more effectively regardless of parental anatomy.

Nursing bras. A must-have, but wait until the baby is here! If you are sizing out of all your bras, go ahead and replace them with soft bras that can be pulled up and down as needed, but don't invest much money in this phase. Over the first six weeks, your body will change dramatically and then settle at a more stable size. That is the right time to buy nicer nursing bras. What you need for the early weeks are nursing camisoles or sleep bras that are good for home and have some stretch. If you need more support than that, buy some less-expensive nursing bras for the time being. You can find these at local specialty baby/parent retailers, online, or at any big box store.

Milk storage bags. These are a really efficient way to store milk. They are also available at most drug and grocery stores, so you don't need them ahead of time.

A pump or a plan to rent one, if needed. I do know people in this day and age who never pumped, but most of us end up expressing milk at some point. If you are on the fence, you can rent a pump or pick one up at Target if you need one last minute, but I think they are good to have pre-baby in case you run into trouble and need to have it to maintain milk production. Just leave it in the box and return it if you don't use it. You can also choose to exclusively hand express (see page 160 for an explanation of this). This can have a bit of a learning curve but can be really effective. Think of it as more tools in your toolbox: maybe you'll find you love it, maybe you'll only use it in a pinch.

Bottles and bottle brush. Even if you don't plan to use bottles, it's good to be prepared. Refer to the bottle section for more advice on how to choose a bottle. Bottle brushes are essential for cleaning pumps, but they can get funky, so I recommend buying an inexpensive one and replacing it every few months.

Maybe have

Breast shells. These are to help with soreness or leaking and range from a little globe that keeps fabric up off your nipple to silver disks or natural seashells. While there is no particular research to support these, they can be an excellent defence against babies, toddlers, or cats brushing up against sore nipples.

Hydrogels. These are almost a hybrid between a breast shell and a nipple cream. They provide moist wound healing to help nipples heal after a bad latch, as well as protect your nipples from clothes or being bumped by the dog.

Nursing pads. Almost no one needs these right away, but after your milk transition, things can get a little leaky. Disposable or reusable nursing pads help keep your clothes and bed dry.

Passive milk collection pump or hand pump passive collection pump: These cheap silicon bulbs catch extra milk while nursing or can work as a hand pump in a power outage, or they can be good just to have in your bag in case your meeting runs long. A true hand pump has more parts to it but also allows you to control suction a little better. These two items are fairly interchangeable and very helpful.

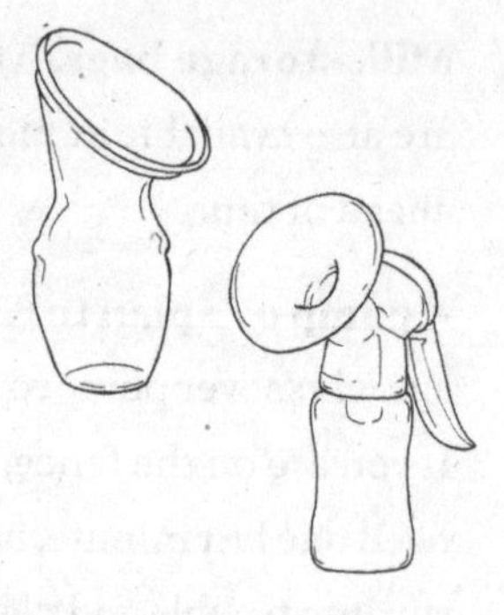

Don't need

Nursing covers. Some people feel more private about nursing than others. In general, you can use a scarf or a blanket to give yourself some privacy. Dedicated nursing covers do have extra features that make them easier to use. If it sounds like something you would use often, then it might be worth it, but most people don't need one.

Bottle trial kits. Instead, just start with a good bottle (page 138), introduce it between two and six weeks (see page 202 for how to do this), and you will be unlikely to find yourself needing to try different bottles.

We'll get into exactly how to nurse, from first latch to ongoing challenges, later in the book (see page 89). Most parents do some amount of bottle feeding. Whether pumped milk or formula, refer to the next sections for an overview of what's involved and what you'll need.

BOTTLE FEEDING

Whether you're planning to exclusively bottle feed from birth (formula, pumped or donor milk), are wondering about combining nursing and bottle feeding, or plan to supplement nursing with pumped milk, here's what to bear in mind.

PROS

Bonding and help. Bottles are an awesome tool for spreading the work around. Anyone can learn to "paced bottle feed" (page 144), and families or caregivers sharing this role is a great fit for some families. It is also just very bonding to feed babies. More people getting to feed the baby makes everyone feel close and connected.

Bottles are pretty easy to come by. They sell them lots of places, they aren't particularly expensive, and while some are better than others (page 203), any bottle will work in a pinch.

CONS

Supply chains. Something has to go into bottles. This can be milk you pump, milk someone else pumps, or formula from the store. These are all good options, but drops in personal production, drops in donor milk supply, or formula recalls and shortages can be stressful.

A little more work than direct nursing. In the middle of the night, preparing a bottle is a little bit more work that nursing. That being said, it's not prohibitively hard, and you didn't get into parenting thinking it would be easy.

Some small health risks. In large-scale studies there is a slightly higher instance of eczema and GI infections in formula-fed babies. Person to person, I don't think the risks outweigh the benefits to most families.

WHAT YOU'LL NEED

There are a lot of bottles and bottle accessories out there. Bottle feeding can be a fairly minimalist affair. Some basic items that you will need, and likely already have:

- Hot water
- A mug
- Clean water
- Dish soap
- 5–10 towels and small blankets for rolling and positioning
- 2–4 extra pillows. You can get a dedicated infant-feeding pillow or just use pillows from around the house.

What you'll need to buy

Two to four small bottles. I recommend four-ounce narrow-neck bottles with a slow flow or preemie nipple. See page 203 for how to choose.

If you plan on pumping, a pump. I recommend a cordless hospital-grade pump (see page 40 for more discussion of this).

If you are formula feeding. You will be sent home from a hospital birth with enough formula to get you going and you can pick some up at the store, but it's a good idea to have some ready at home. I recommend starting newborns with a partially hydrolyzed formula that is easy to find at a local store. There's more information on choosing a formula and understanding its ingredients on page 77.

An inexpensive bottle brush. Replace it every few months.

Formula containers. The ability to mix bottles on the go is crucial. These containers have separate chambers to hold the right number of scoops for your baby's bottle. You prefill it and then you just need to bring a bottle of water and baby bottle when you go out.

Maybe have

Bottle warmer. Many babies aren't picky about cold or room temperature bottles, and plopping a bottle into a mug of hot water will do the trick to warm it up. However, if you like gadgets and have the counter space, go to town. There are many of these on the market. You will need to get to know the settings on your specific bottle warmer very well and must always test bottles for temperature. Swirl warmed milk and put a few drops on your wrist. It should feel warm but not hot. Do not microwave bottles of milk or formula, only the water you use to warm them in. Microwaves don't heat consistently, causing hot spots in milk that can burn a baby.

Coolers and cool storage. If you live in a warm climate, this is a great way to keep milk cold while on the go. My favorites are lunch boxes that can be frozen or have a built-in freezer bag.

Thermos. A way to keep water warm for mixing or warming bottles when out and about can be very handy. Alternately, you can put coffee in it.

Don't need

Drying racks. If you are a very clean person, you are allowed to have one of these, and it must be cleaned at least once a week. If, like me, you have never in your life even thought about washing your dish rack, I recommend a clean dish towel with a paper towel on top of it.

Formula mixing machine. Formula is instant. You don't need to brew it or make it. These machines are likely to trap old formula or mold unless they are fully disassembled and cleaned once a week, which is more trouble than it's worth. They can also be inaccurate in how they mix formula which can be dangerous to babies who are gaining weight slowly.

Sterilizers. Infant feeding is food prep, not surgery. In the US, unless your baby is medically fragile and sterilized formula and feeding supplies are recommended by your pediatrician, there is no need/point to sterilizing bottles and/or pump parts. Breast milk isn't sterile, home-mixed formula isn't sterile, none of the food you eat is sterile. So, you can go ahead and think of pump supplies and bottles the same way you do plates: wash them in warm soapy water, and you are good to go.

So, you have your shopping list. Now what? We'll get into how to choose a bottle and nipples, as well as exactly how to bottle feed a baby, on page 203.

PARTNERS

It's common for partners and non-nursing parents to make bottle feeding "their zone." If you are exclusively bottle feeding your baby, then you can divide the labor up however makes sense. There is no reason for you not to become a bottle-feeding expert. I have seen some co-parents really master paced bottle feeding and put me to shame. A little tip: Choose a feeding every day that is your feeding. That way your partner can predictably plan on stepping away and getting a break at that time.

PUMPING

You may know that you will need to—or think you want to—exclusively pump from the beginning. You may be expecting a baby who will need to go to the NICU for medical care, or you might want to give your baby your milk, but bottle feeding is a better fit. If you are nursing, chances are that, at some point, you will also find yourself pumping, so it's worth finding out what's involved and what you will need in advance.

PROS

Autonomy. Pumping allows you to control when, how, and how long you express milk, instead of feeding on demand.

Human milk feeding during separation. Whether your baby needs to be separated from you for medical, work, or fun reasons, pumping allows us to provide milk while we are away.

Jumpstarting milk production if your baby isn't ready. Whether due to prematurity, illness, tongue-tie, or just plain learning, pumping is a good way to build a milk supply while your baby or babies work on nursing skills.

Stashing milk. Some people with a high production can pump a few times a day or for a few months and provide enough milk to bottle feed their baby and meet their goals. Some people find that they are able to make a large milk supply with the reliable stimulation of modern pumps. This is a body thing, not a skill thing. You will need to follow your body's lead and see if this is a good fit for you.

Inducing lactation. You don't need to birth a baby to make milk. Pumping is a great tool for non-gestational parents to start making milk to feed to their babies without having a pregnancy. If you did not birth your baby but have breasts, you can use pumping to tell your body to make milk. Most protocols begin with hormones to simulate a pregnancy followed by pumping, but you can also just pump, and eventually your body will begin making milk.

CONS

Hard to do in public. While nursing in public is accepted more and more, public pumping isn't, and if I'm being honest, this is probably because it's a lot of nipple in a way nursing isn't. This is improving with more in-bra pump options.

Difficult to maintain. If you are only pumping and aim to produce all the food your baby needs, most people would need to pump 8–10 times per day for 10–30 minutes in the beginning; that is a lot of set up and time to figure out on top of the rest of your life. I found it annoying and frustrating, and many people just don't like pumping very much. This is extremely subjective, and you should feel good about following the pumping path that feels right to you.

WHAT YOU'LL NEED

Must have

Pump(s). See below for a guide on how to choose.

Pumping bras. These are bras or bandeaux that hold a pump in place. This leaves your hands free for massage, snacking, or emailing. If you plan to exclusively pump from the beginning, get a very adjustable and sturdy bra first. The wrap around bandeau style with a Velcro back is a great option. You do not yet know what size you will be, and this way you can diversify after six weeks, when you have a better sense of the big picture.

Pump parts. Pump parts are hard to source ahead of time because they need to be sized, and pumping before birth can induce premature labor. Most pumps come with a few sizes, but you may be outside that size range. A lactation consultant should be able to fit you with the right size, or you can order multiple sizes and use trial and error. Once you know your size, you can start customising, add a second, more portable pump, and get extras of parts you might want as backup. If your baby is already here or you are inducing lactation without pregnancy, go to the guide to flange fit on page 155 to assess if we can already determine that you will need a bigger or smaller flange.

Maybe have

Pump bag. If you are going to be traveling out and back to work, a pumping bag can be a nice way to stay organized and clean. However, you can absolutely just use a bag you already have and a lunch box.

Don't need

Sterilizers. Again, infant feeding is food prep, not surgery. You can go ahead and think of pump supplies (and bottles) as you would plates: wash them in warm soapy water, and you are good to go.

CHOOSING A PUMP

New pumps come out all the time, so I'll speak generally in case new models have been released since the date I'm writing this.

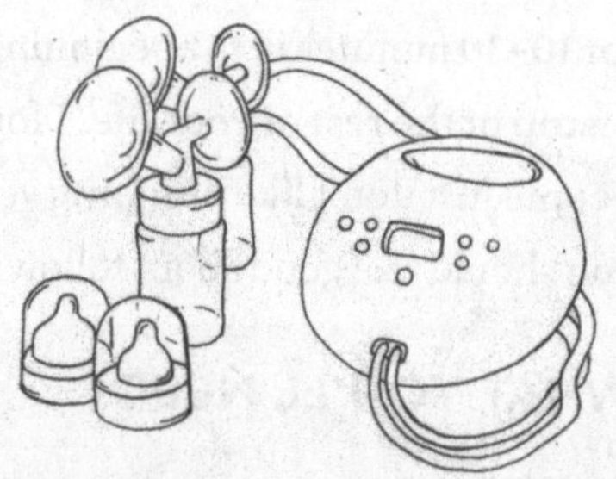

Hospital grade vs. single user

I recommend ordering a "hospital-grade pump" if your insurance offers that option, as they tend to work better and last longer. Hospital-grade pumps can be shared or handed down. That means they have a closed system and no milk can get inside and make a moldy mess. They also have a longer motor life. Some hospital-grade pumps are large and impractical, not to mention expensive, but your workplace may offer one in a designated pumping room, and most hospitals have them for use postpartum or in the NICU. These larger hospital-grade pumps can also be rented. You may be able to find a closed system personal pump at a secondhand store or website; just wash any of the bottles and flanges when it comes to you.

There are also smaller hospital-grade pumps that are covered by insurance. I recommend getting one of these. My current favorite is the Spectra S1.

Single-user pumps are designed to be safely used by one person for roughly 2.5 kids' worth of motor. I don't recommend these because they tend to be less customizable and due to the fact that they are single-user, which means that they cannot be donated and reused, which is a landfill problem. These are not my preferred pumps, but if that is all you have access to in your area or in your budget, they will work just fine.

Cordless vs. corded

I recommend getting a cordless pump. In the age of smartphones, the idea that you need to be within 3 feet of an outlet for half your day is maddening, so if you can make the price difference work, free yourself. If your insurance company covers a pump, you may be able to find a durable medical equipment company that lets you pay the difference to upgrade to a cordless pump.

In-bra pumps

These fit entirely into a bra, and some of them even make pumping laying down possible. There are also accessories you can add to other pumps to be able to keep your top on while pumping, but attached to an external machine.

These pumps are extremely convenient, and often expensive. They also don't have a wide range of suction and lack the adjustability of a traditional pump, so I recommend starting use of these pumps after six weeks. I also recommend getting a more traditional pump to start in order to figure out what you need in terms of milk-holding capacity and flange size. Flanges for in-bra pumps are sometimes sized very differently from other pumps because they use continuous

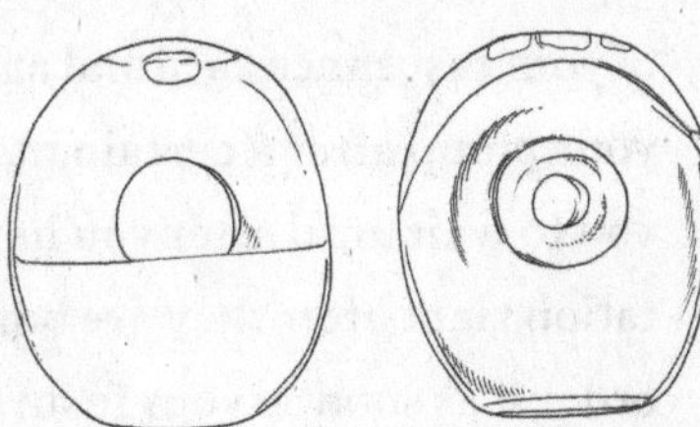

suction instead of intermittent suction. I highly recommend you find online groups of people using these in-bra pumps for directions on sizing.

If this is not your first baby, and you know more about your preferred suction levels and flange fit, you can use this information to chose a more portable pump that is specific to your needs as your main pump this time.

A few other variables to consider when choosing a pump

Are you often on work calls? Check reviews and invest in something quiet.

Is there a multiuser pump that stays at work provided by your workplace? Consider buying the same brand so your parts are interchangeable.

HOW TO ORDER A PUMP THROUGH INSURANCE

If you have Medicaid, then you qualify for a program called Women, Infants, and Children (WIC). They provide food assistance and lactation help to families who receive Medicaid. Remember that the Medicaid threshold changes significantly once you have a baby to include a larger income range, so you if you didn't qualify before, it may be worth checking again. Their peer counselors and lactation teams are truly excellent, and I learned much of what is in this book from the time I spent in WIC offices. You should absolutely use this resource if it is available to you. Access to pumps varies somewhat from county to county, but go ahead and reach out to the WIC office to understand their policy and get connected with their team.

With the passage of the Affordable Care Act, most American insurance plans now cover breast pumps. If you have a private insurer, you should ask them what their specific protocol for ordering a pump is. In most cases, your birthing provider will write you a prescription and your insurance company will recommend a provider of "durable medical equipment" or a DME. The best way to get this information is to call the number on the back of your insurance card and ask. Some insurance companies have you order your pump after a certain number of weeks of pregnancy; others require you to wait until after you have your baby. If your baby needs supplementation right after they are born, having a pump around would be good, so order it as soon as your insurance allows. If they require you to wait until after your baby is born, don't worry: your birthing place will have pumps for you to use, and in many cases will allow you to rent them. The worst-case scenario is that you will spend $150 on one that gets delivered to your house within an hour from a big box store, or call your local WIC office who will provide you with a pump. You can also safely borrow a pump from a friend while you wait for yours to come.

Some plans were able to avoid new regulation by the ACA and do not cover pumps. If that is the case, you will need to buy a pump yourself. On the scale of medical equipment, they are not very expensive, but you can absolutely wait until you need one to purchase one. Previously used pumps can also be bought secondhand and you only need to purchase or wash the flanges and bottles. This is a great choice both financially and environmentally.

CHAPTER 3

WHAT ELSE TO CONSIDER

Now that you have an overview of each type of feeding, it's helpful to dig deeper into what feeding styles are the best fit for your family and situation. Your range of choices and things to consider may be influenced by how your baby will come into your life.

BIRTHING

If you or your partner is giving birth to your baby, you can breastfeed or offer bottles of formula, donor milk, or your pumped milk.

ADOPTION

Depending on the style of adoption you have and your relationship with the birth parents in your triad, you may have a few different feeding options. It is most common to feed adopted babies formula or donor milk. You can also induce lactation in your own body and breastfeed an adopted baby, though you should know that if infertility brought you to adoption, some of the factors that cause infertility can also cause low milk production, so check out the anatomy section of this book (page 89) to see if this is a good option for you.

Adoption is complex, and adopting parents should remember that birth parents are an important part of your triad and respect their autonomy in how the baby is fed during this transitional time. If your placement comes after a baby is born or very close to birth, you may not have time to make careful plans and will likely use formula or donor milk initially. You can induce lactation over your first few months together if that feels right to you.

If you are a birth mother or birth parent considering an adoption plan, you can nurse your baby or plan to bottle feed your baby before placement. Some people find it healing and positive to donate milk as part of an open adoption, some don't. Remember that regardless of your placement plan, those early moments and days are for you, and you are entitled during them to feed your baby however feels right. That may be you or your family feeding your baby, it may also be having the intended family do the feeding. It is your choice.

FOSTER CARE

Parenting through foster care gives parents the least choice in how their babies are fed. If you are in the US, your formula costs will be covered at least in part by your baby's food assistance program. It is not legal to breastfeed or feed donor milk to your baby in this case because their medical decisions involve the state. The one exception to this is premature babies, who may be given donor milk prescribed by their doctor while in the NICU. You can advocate for what feels best to you with your baby's medical team and legal decision-makers.

SURROGACY

You may decide to offer bottles of formula or donor milk from birth. You may also negotiate into your surrogacy agreement a certain amount of time that you would like to ask your surrogate to pump milk for your baby. You can also find friends or community donors who will pump milk for your baby. You may want to have conversations with your surrogate about what feels right about bottles/ breastfeeding while all in the hospital together. If you have breasts, it is also an option for you to induce lactation.

YOUR BABY'S BODY

Babies are born with their own personalities and their own body differences. Babies are individuals and it's best to treat them that way. A variable that is largely out of your control is your baby's body. Whether due to disability, prematurity, asymmetry or oral ties: babies come with their own stuff. I cannot cover every way that baby's bodies impact how they eat, but I will focus on the two most common ones: oral ties and positional asymmetries.

ORAL TIES (ANKYLOGLOSSIA)

A "tie" is a tight piece of tissue that connects the tongue or lip to the mouth in a way that restricts functional movement.

What are the different types of ties?

Open your mouth as wide as you can. Without moving your jaw up, can you reach your tongue to the roof of your mouth? Using your fingers, can you lift your top lip up over your nostrils?

If you do this in a mirror you will notice little attachment points between your tongue and the floor of your mouth, and your upper lip and gums. These are called frenulums or frenums.

- Tongue-tie is a tight lingual frenulum
- Lip-tie is a tight labial frenulum (note that only the top lip is relevant here)

In utero, babies' tongues and lips are fully attached to the gum ridge with collagen. Then as they develop, the cells at these attachment points mostly die off, leaving a smaller, more flexible attachment. In some babies, however, the cells don't die off or the tissue is made of a different collagen that doesn't stretch. Both are genetic. If ties have been spotted elsewhere in your baby's genetic family (genetic parent or sibling) it is worth having your baby assessed.

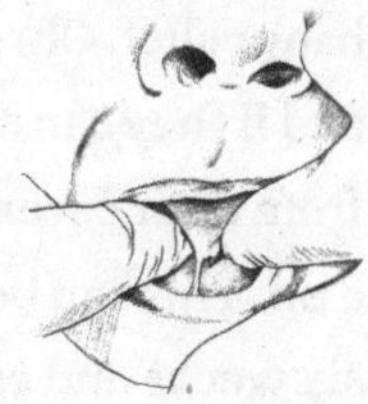

Tongue-ties can look all kinds of ways. Some ties attach all the way to the tip of the tongue and give the tongue a heart-shaped appearance. They can also start farther back and be relatively short, or not look tied but have no stretch.

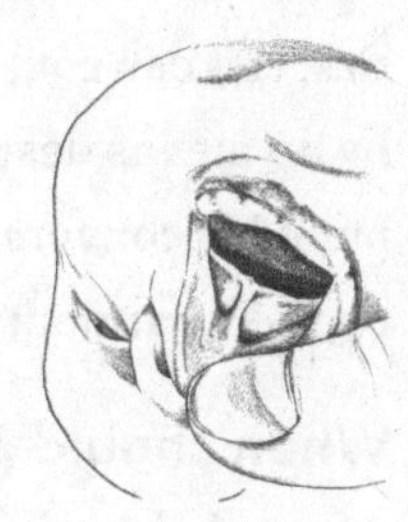

Lip-ties. A lip tie is an attachment from the top lip to the gums. You can do a simple check by lifting your baby's lip up all the way over their nostrils. Did their gums or frenulum turn white from the stretch?

Lip- and tongue-ties are common and usually come together.

Buccal-ties are attachments between the gums and cheeks. While these kinds of ties can occur and can affect feeding, they are much rarer than tongue-ties and lip-ties and many providers prefer to leave them alone.

Signs of a tie

- Pain while nursing
- Nipple of bottle or breast comes out of baby's mouth compressed
- Uncomfortable gas
- Reflux
- White tongue; buildup isn't cleared by the roof of the mouth
- Difficulty gaining weight
- Very frequent feedings
- Slow to eat bottles
- Tongue staying low in mouth during crying
- Difficulty relaxing shoulders
- Mouth breathing
- Snoring
- Sleeping with an open mouth

If your baby has these symptoms, it is worth seeking out an assessment to see if a revision (a procedure to cut this tissue) might give you or your baby relief. Chronic nursing pain and colicky babies are just horrendous, and if they can be resolved they should. Some babies can easily eat enough from their parent's letdown and never actually engage a strong suck due to a tie. This can be very challenging when milk production changes around six weeks and can result in a drop in production. Beyond feeding difficulties, ties can cause difficulties with speech or sleep down the road. This is by no means destiny, and we do not treat all tongue-ties prophylactically, but it is a conversation worth having with your diagnosing provider. More on the treatment and aftercare of ties on pages 49–50.

When should a tie be revised?

After a baby is born a pediatrician, midwife, nurse or lactation consultant may screen for tongue-ties. If a baby has a very obvious tie they may treat it with surgical scissors in the days shortly after birth. For most babies, however, a tie is too hard to spot at this age as it is usually hidden by the bunched muscles and recessed jaw of newborns. If a tongue-tie is spotted soon after birth and the medical team feels good about treating it you should do so, but know that your baby may need a second procedure between two and twelve weeks, when the jaw has more fully developed and the full frenulum is visible.

Optimally, tongue-ties are treated between two and six weeks. This is when babies are developed enough that a provider can get good access to the tie, but not so late that its likely to have impacted milk production. After six months many providers would recommend anaesthesia for a release which opens a new set of risk benefits calculations.

Many parents find the fact that one provider may suspect a tie and others don't frustrating and confusing. This variation in opinion usually has more to do with the timing of the assessment and the experience/lens of the practitioner than the tie itself. You may suspect a missed tie if you are in constant pain with nursing that isn't resolving with improving your latch, or a baby isn't gaining weight well or is very gassy/burps often.

Is it a yeast infection or a tie?

Babies' mouths (just like adult mouths) are full of a healthy microbiome that helps digest food, keep mouths clean, and is part of the immune system.

Sometimes this microbiome (just like any other in the body) can get out of balance. The most common of these imbalances is a yeast overgrowth. Babies who have had antibiotics are at higher risk for a yeast infection in their mouth. There was a time when we thought that these yeast infections could easily transfer to the ducts of the nursing parent causing pain and infection. Yeast on parent's nipples was a very common diagnosis in the past, and still is in some practices. It is not however well backed up by science. We often find that what is called "nipple thrush" is actually nerve damage from a bad latch/tongue-tie or vasospasm. Yeast infections in and on breasts is actually very rare, and if you suspect one, you should have a culture taken to make sure you are treating the real cause of your pain (see page 49 on skin and ductal yeast). Ask your provider to do a culture from your nipple to confirm yeast before treating it.

Yeast in babies' mouths shows up as big, thick patches of white surrounded by redness on the gums, the roof of the mouth, and the inside of a baby's cheeks. These yeast infections can result in a baby using their mouth differently in a way that can cause pain for a nursing person.

Yeast infections do not look like whiteness on a baby's tongue. This is a sign that a baby has a vaulted palate or tongue-tie, resulting in an inability to rub the tongue on the roof of the mouth and clean it.

Tongue-tie treatment

To treat a tie, the cartilage is cut with either surgical scissors or a laser. The different tools have pros and cons. I prefer to go with the tool your local provider feels most comfortable using, rather than focusing on the tool itself. If the provider who is recommended in your area uses a specific tool that is different from what was used by a friend in another town, that is okay. What is essential is that the provider has a lot of training in the tool they are using.

WHAT TO EXPECT AT A FRENOTOMY APPOINTMENT

If you or one of your providers suspects that your baby has a tie and they could benefit functionally from a frenotomy, you'll be referred to a clinic for assessment and treatment. Most places offer both in the same visit if it is indicated, but you can always ask to split assessment and treatment into two visits so you have time to think and decide.

SUCK EXAM AND ORAL REVIEW OF CIRCUMSTANCES

Your clinician should do a thorough functional exam and ask lots of questions about what is going on. This assures you that there is a functional issue, not just the appearance of a tie.

PROCEDURE

The actual procedure is very quick. In some clinics you will stay with your baby; in others, they will take your baby away for a short time to do the procedure. Babies do not need anesthesia for the procedure. It is painful, but very quick. Babies tend to cry similarly to being vaccinated. The clinician will cut the tissue with a laser or scissors and then observe for bleeding. If there is bleeding, they will hold pressure on the site until it clots. Another way to hold pressure on the tissue is to nurse, so some providers prefer this option. This is more common with a scissor procedure than a laser procedure. Don't be alarmed if this is suggested by your provider, but it is a good idea to ask what to expect after the procedure when you arrive for assessment.

FEEDING/SNUGGLES FOR COMFORT

After release, your baby may immediately eat or suck for comfort. Sucking is extremely effective at baby pain management, though you can also talk to your pediatrician about giving your baby Tylenol or ibuprofen before the procedure to help with pain.

AFTERCARE

Your provider will give your baby specific stretches and exercises to make sure that the site heals well. Mouths heal very quickly because they have so much blood flow, and so frenula can reattach if you don't take care to hold them open. If you've ever had a piercing, this is similar, where you need to keep the site open until it heals so that it doesn't heal closed. This usually consists of lifting the tongue up for 30 seconds at diaper changes or before feedings but may include different stretches or exercises depending on the tool your provider used and your baby's specific circumstances.

This is what a tie would look like before and after a procedure.

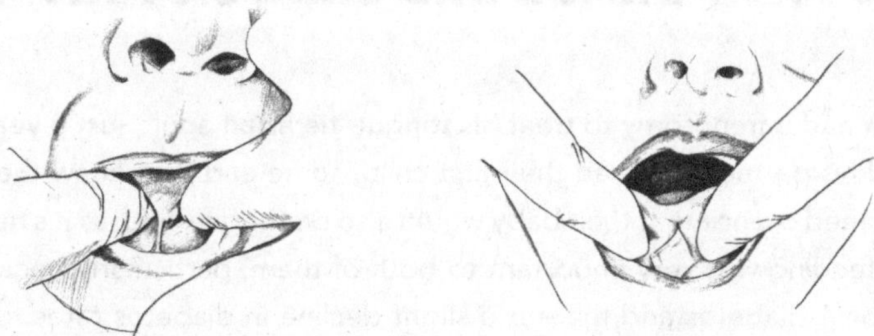

Suck training

We think babies are brand-new at birth, but remember, they have been sucking and swallowing since about fifteen weeks' gestation. That means that they have a lot of habits around how they have learned to suck. In my experience, about half of babies immediately eat better after a revision and about half need extra help from a lactation/feeding professional to learn a new suck pattern. This usually includes tummy time and lots of tug of war with breast or bottle to build up coordination and strength with the correct muscles. Babies who have ties still have a drive to eat and may suck harder, not smarter. They often have a very strong suck using the cheek or neck muscles to make up for their restricted tongue or lips. Teaching a baby to use the correct muscles can take some time but should get better. You can rest assured that if your baby is needing this extra help to relearn sucking, you did the right thing getting a release. These are likely the kids whom we would see for speech or respiratory issues down the road if left untreated. You can reach out to a speech therapist who is experienced with babies or a lactation professional to get guidance on how to strengthen and teach good sucking techniques.

My baby has a tie but eats just fine

Do I have to do anything about it? Nope. But I would keep an eye on it and grab a six-week weight check if you are nursing. Some babies are able to rely on their parent's flow until six weeks and then will drop weight because they can't maintain it on their own.

DAMON AND SARA'S STORY

Damon had a frenotomy to treat his tongue-tie as an adult, just a year before he and his partner Sara had their first child, so he and Sara knew there was a heightened chance that their baby would also be tongue-tied, as it's hereditary. Breastfeeding was very important to both of them, particularly because Sara has type 1 diabetes and there is a slight decline in diabetes rates for babies who are breast-fed. Between those two concerns, both of them were on the lookout for signs of tongue-tie.

After Simone was born, though, the breastfeeding went well. Sara had a generous milk supply, Simone was growing well, and Sara wasn't particularly in pain. They were still concerned, however. They factored in that often if a tongue-tied baby isn't doing the work to draw milk and stimulate the nursing person's hormones, their milk supply can decline over time.

Even with the family history, it took eight weeks to get a definitive answer on whether there was tongue-tie, and if the procedure was medically necessary. Damon had a long struggle with neck pain and sleep apnea due to the condition and knew that the impacts of the tie could be long lasting, so when they found out that Simone was a candidate, they decided to move forward. Because of his own experience, Damon knew that the procedure would hurt, and the aftercare would, too.

Once the surgery was complete, Damon was in charge of lifting Simone's tongue so that the site didn't close right back. "I didn't want to complicate things by having Sara be the one to cause Simone pain [by sweeping Simone's mouth to make sure the tie didn't reattach]. But it sucked for me to be going in her mouth four times a day and making her cry." He also felt genetic shame that he was the one who had passed the tongue-tie on to her.

At Simone's follow up visit, the dentist manually reopened the incision, which had begun to close slightly. More guilt for Damon, who felt as though this, too, was his fault for not doing the sweeps hard enough. However, three days later he noticed that his daughter's range of motion in her neck had totally changed. The revision had not only improved her nursing but had impacted her gross motor abilities. "I really don't have any regrets. For a while, I was on the lookout for lasting trauma or distress, but there wasn't any." For their family, releasing the tongue-tie despite mixed messages from providers was absolutely the right decision.

UNDERSTANDING BABY ALIGNMENT

A close cousin of the tongue tie is what is called: positional asymmetries. This is another kind of tightness that can impact a baby's eating and development. Babies grow in a very compact space, and are designed to be born from an even more compact space. To accommodate this, the bones of a baby's head are made to bend and overlap. Maybe you noticed after your baby was born how perfectly round, or cone headed, their head was based on their presentation and birth.

If your baby wasn't perfectly aligned in the birth canal, or got a bit squished on the way out (this can happen with vaginal or cesarean births), then there is a mechanism to pull things back into place. That mechanism is eating. The muscles around the mouth and face are connected to the plates of the skull and bones of the neck. As these muscles get stronger through eating, babies' faces and heads change shape. If a baby is too crunched to eat effectively, or has an oral tie that prevents them from using the correct muscles, this realignment can't happen.

While this smooshed head situation is very cool design, nature is never perfect, and all bodies are different. Sometimes one of the plates of the skull overlaps another and cannot be moved back with feeding alone; in these cases, a bodyworker (massage therapist, osteopath or chiropractor) or physical therapist can gently assist your baby in moving it into place.

Parents of multiples should note that your babies may need extra attention in this area, because they are more likely to have difficult asymmetries due to being most squished in utero.[1]

These asymmetries and misalignments are common and are one of the leading causes of breastfeeding pain beyond a shallow latch. Most parents—and, honestly, pediatricians—don't notice these small differences, but they can make a big impact. They are foundational, meaning that what is very small now can become much larger later. The earlier these issues are addressed, the easier they are to work on. For instance, a small head turning preference as a six-week-old can become a flat spot at six months and an asymmetrical crawl at nine months, which both take much more effort to correct.

I want you to imagine a very long car ride. You get out at the gas station, and you need to streeeeetch. Do it with me right now: Stretch your arms out wide and your head back. That feels pretty good for most humans, since we are a slouchy bunch.

Now imagine you get from that car directly into a hammock. Then into an egg chair. Then a squishy couch. You never get a chance to stretch out, as you are still always curled into a C-shape.

Your baby just completed a nine-month car ride, and they need a chance to stretch. You'll notice most of our baby tools (car seats, swaddles, wraps, swings) keep baby in that curled-up position. That is fine; babies like these tools because they remind them of being in utero, and tools are great, but like a good yoga teacher, I want you to be mindful of offering opportunities for a counter-stretch.

Fascia is a network of fibers that encase every muscle and organ in the body. Fascia is like an elaborate tension system that keeps everything it its place. It can also bunch in a certain area, causing what people think of as a "knot" in a muscle.

Imagine setting up a tent. As you use tension to balance the tent up, pulling too hard in one direction will pull the whole tent down. When it bunches in one direction, it throws the network of stakes and poles out of alignment. Some areas are too loose; others are too tight. To help fascia un-bunch we use heat and time. The heat of your hands is a great tool for sensitive little babies. If you notice that your baby is holding tension, you can simply place your hand on that spot and hold it there with just the smallest amount of pressure, like you are sliding a piece of paper across a table, and as the fascia warms from your hand, it will start to release. There is actually one long line of fascia that connects your tongue to your toes. This is one of the ways feeding impacts the whole body. The most likely area of tension that parents spot is babies who keep one shoulder close to their ear. Try using the weight of your hand and the warmth of it resting on your baby's shoulder to help them relax those muscles.

For most babies, simple stretches, tummy time, and eating are enough to sort out any issues. If you or your baby is in consistent pain, or you are noticing that they are out of alignment after the three-week mark, it may be a good idea to get some extra help on board.

TRY A BATH

Baths are so good for bonding and realigning. The change of gravity and the warmth of the water can help your baby hold their own body in positions they find comfortable. Draw a warm bath, though likely cooler than you would have it for just yourself, and try unwinding or just snuggling in the bath. Follow your baby's lead and let them find comfortable positions in their body. This is a great non-birthing parent activity if birth recovery means a parent cannot yet soak.

Two things to be specifically aware of in your baby's body are torticollis and plagiocephaly.

Torticollis is tension in one side of your baby's body that causes them to have difficulty moving their head equally in both directions. This can cause pain for a baby or pain for the nursing parent. Think of yourself with a strained muscle in your calf walking up the stairs. You may hold on extra tight to the banister. Some babies compensate for tightness or discomfort by chewing instead of sucking—this is a common source of nursing pain or dysfunctional bottle eating.

Plagiocephaly is known more widely as "flat head." It is often blamed on pressure on flat surfaces or babies sleeping on their backs, but it is actually caused by the inability of the back and neck muscles to pull the head plates back into place.

Depending on severity, these can be corrected between three and nine months with physical therapy and helmeting, but they are both much more easily resolved in the early days of your baby's development. These issues are fairly common, and most people don't even notice them, but if you catch them early, they may help you avoid other interventions later.

The role of the pediatrician on your team is to make sure your baby is growing well, to give you information about and access to vaccinations, and to help refer you to specialists as needed by tracking your baby's development. They are very good at normalizing and telling parents to "wait and see," which is a great approach. That is their role on the team.

They do not spend very much time with your baby and may be less tuned in to your baby's body movement than you. I recommend assessing your baby's alignment yourself and letting your medical team know if you are noticing any patterns that concern you.

Checking your baby's alignment

Signs that you should look into your baby's alignment:

- Burping after every feeding, which may be a sign of swallowing air from an uncoordinated suck
- Baby seems to be in pain
- Baby tends to look in one direction
- Difficulty getting baby to latch to breast or bottle
- Pain while nursing

Look at their face

Your baby is so cute, but let's take a second to look beyond that unbearable adorableness to where everything is on their face. Is one eyebrow higher than the other? Is there a slant to their forehead? Can you see any flat spots on their head?

If you do notice some facial asymmetries, consider that they may be causing nursing pain or could cause some difficulties down the road. There is nothing wrong with your baby; they were squished in the pregnancy or birth process and may need a little extra help getting comfortable and correctly aligned. If you notice good facial alignment, any issues they and their parent might be having are probably unrelated to alignment.

Look at your baby's rolls

A very simple way to see if you should follow up about your baby's alignment is to count their rolls. Lay your baby down in just a diaper and count how many creases there are on their body. Some babies are slimmer and don't have many rolls; that's fine. What we are looking for here is: Are there the same number on each of your baby's arms? Roll them over onto their tummy: Does their back look straight? How many rolls are on the backs of their legs? Is there the same number on each leg?

Look at your camera roll

I know how many photos you have of your baby. How could you not? Take a moment to look through them. Does your baby tend to be looking one way in most photos? Do you always hold them in the same position? Does your baby seem to hold their body in a curve?

Where to find help

It is sometimes the case that babies need help beyond at-home stretches and tummy time. If you or your baby is in consistent pain or you are noticing persistent asymmetry, I recommend checking in with one of the following providers.

INFANT BODYWORK

Assuming you had just had a nine-month car ride, you might also find yourself in need of a massage. Infant bodywork can be done by a massage therapist, an osteopath, or a chiropractor. It is very different from some adult bodywork in that babies' bodies need very little pressure to help guide them into the right position. Infant bodyworkers use about the same amount of pressure you would use if you were checking if a tomato is ripe. Infant massage and chiropractic care look very different from their adult counterparts. Look for someone who specializes in infants and ask about their training specifically for babies.

One Canadian study conducted a controlled trial where an osteopath did real bodywork on some babies and fake body work on others. The researchers found that infants who received real bodywork had better latches. This is because misalignment and nerve impingement can cause a baby to have an uncoordinated suck or a chewing motion that can cause pain.[2]

INFANT PHYSICAL THERAPY

Another option is to see a physical therapist. Some physical therapists use manual therapy like a bodyworker, but most will assess your baby's range of motion and give you specific tools and exercises to address this. You may need a referral from your pediatrician for your insurance to cover this option—call your insurance company directly and ask. Look for someone who specializes in babies, as they even sometimes make house calls.

TUMMY TIME

Tummy time can feel extremely pointless, as few practitioners take the time to explain why we do it. It also tends to make babies mad (because it is hard), and we don't like to make babies mad, especially in the very few awake minutes they have in a day. Tummy time can start as soon as a baby is born. In the early days it is easiest to do with an awake baby held chest to chest by a parent or caregiver lying flat on their back. As they get a little older (two weeks and beyond), you'll add a roll in and out of tummy time to increase range of motion and build strength.

The best way to realign the plates of a baby's skull after birth is by having a baby use their back and neck muscles to pull them into alignment through baby push-ups, i.e., tummy time.

If you ask any physical therapist how much time a baby should spend on their tummy, they will say half their waking time. So somewhere between five and five thousand minutes per day, depending on your baby. I find this recommendation unhelpful, so here are some tummy-time tips I have found to actually help, through working alongside brilliant bodyworker and illustrator Ayden Love:

- Reps not duration: This is your baby's gym time. It is not about how long they stay in tummy time at one time. It is about how much time they spend in it overall. So, it is much easier to go for more short bursts of tummy time throughout the day than to roll out the Montessori play mat and plan an entire developmental activity that will inevitably go south about five seconds in.

- Find a good time of day for repetition. I find that before diaper changes is a great time to add in some tummy time. You are usually already on a flat surface, and it will only add a few minutes to the diaper change. Babies need changing so often, it adds up to a lot of time throughout your day.
- Roll into tummy time. People are rarely taught the most important part of tummy time: the roll. The roll over the shoulder creates stretch in the neck muscles and gives your baby the very important sensation of how to move their body through space. It also helps them integrate and dampen some of their newborn reflexes, which will help them sleep without a swaddle.

Does babywearing and time on my chest count? Yes and no. These are both great activities for your baby's development. For tummy time on your chest, think of an assisted pull-up bar at the gym. The more upright you are, the more you are assisting your baby in lifting their head. For this reason, they get more credit based on how flat you are. For the highest level of tummy-time success, lie completely flat with your baby on your chest pushing up to look around.

Babywearing is great for babies' hips as well as developing their vestibular system and for back and neck strengthening. It is also giving an alternative to being in a container, which is awesome, but good babywearing won't build strength in the same way as tummy time.

Other ways to let your baby stretch

One of my fundamental rules is: Babies are people, too. No one likes to be stretched beyond their range of motion by another person. It's also not very effective to stretch when you are upset. Your baby will be most responsive to these stretches when they are in their "quiet alert" state (i.e., awake but not mad) and when you let them lead the way.

Unwinding. This is a variation on lifting your baby up like Simba in *The Lion King*, so I recommend doing this sitting on or leaning over your bed for your added security. Cup your baby's bottom in one hand, and place your other hand at the base of your baby's neck. Lift your baby up to your chest level and hold them out in the air like you are presenting them to your kingdom. Now, let your baby lead. You'll notice your baby start to initiate a twist or turn in their body. Your job is not to create any stretch, but rather just to follow and listen.

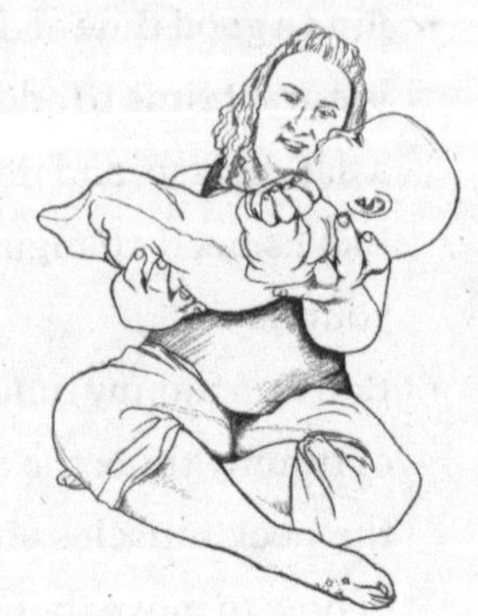

Guppy pose. Begin with one hand cradling your baby's bottom and the other supporting the base of their head at the neck. Follow your baby as they open up their chest and lean back. If your baby does a little crunch inward, that means that the stretch went too far. Come back up to where they were comfortable and let them slowly drop back a little farther. You can also do this by laying your baby across your lap tummy up and cradle the base of their neck in one hand.

You may have noticed guppy pose is upside-down tummy time. Guppy pose gives babies all the range of motion we are looking for from tummy time; it does not, however, give the shoulder flexibility and strength building of tummy time, so try out both.

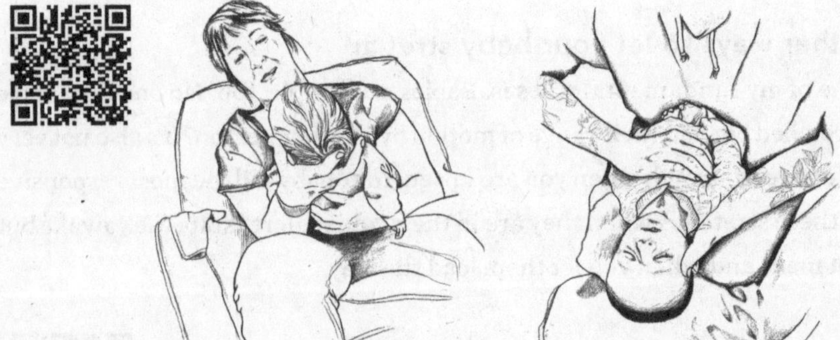

Is this important if I'm bottle feeding or not in pain?

Yes, these issues can affect your child as they grow and develop. Remember that how we feed babies shapes their mouths, builds strength, and lays the foundation for eating solid foods as well as for speech.

Using bottle feeding to help with alignment

Bottle feeding can be an excellent tool to help a baby work through tension. If your baby has a preferred side but can still bottle feed well on the other side, try bottle feeding on their less preferred side or alternating. If you are bottle feeding while your baby is sitting up, try sitting your baby on your lap so that you are on their less preferred side. If their twist is so strong that they cannot eat on one side, feed them on their comfortable side and talk to an infant bodyworker for help.

SECTION TWO

MILK, FORMULA, AND FEEDING METHODS.

CHAPTER 4

WHAT AM I FEEDING MY BABY?

As you navigate making feeding decisions, you will want to know what you are feeding your baby. Babies drink breast milk (parental or donor milk) or formula.

This section will help you learn what human milk is, how it's produced, and how your anatomy and intake can affect feeding your baby from your body. It will also explain how breast milk differs from formula. Remember, in this family, different is not better or worse. While formula is different from breast milk, it is based on human milk and, in my personal read of the research, does a really good job approximating it. Formulas also differ slightly from one another, so you may find that one is easier on your baby's digestion than another. We will cover why this is and how to switch.

Once you know more about what we feed babies, we will get into the *hows*. How to make a bottle, how to express milk, how to latch.

WHY DO WE NEED TO KNOW ABOUT MILK?

Mammals make milk. That and the live birth are sort of what we are known for. We also make milk that is very specific for our babies. Human milk has a whole lot of sugar to grow big brains. Camel milk has so much fat to help camel babies stay hydrated in the desert. Cow's milk has a lot of protein to build big muscles.

This is what's called *species-specific milk*. Similarly, milk made for humans is evolved for humans. It's why we don't give human babies regular cow's milk or DIY formula. To make formula from other mammal species specific to humans, it has to go through a lot of changes, which, luckily, we have figured out how to do and do very well. When we control for access to safe water and access to enough formula, population-wide, we see some slight differences in patterns of babies who are only fed breast milk and babies who are only fed formula. On an individual level, the relative risks in health outcomes of formula vs. breast milk are small: a 9.2% rate of GI infection with breast milk compared to 13.1 % for formula; a 3.3% rate of atopic eczema with breast milk compared to 6.3% rate for formula.[3] This is incredibly difficult to study both ethically and scientifically, but medicine and public health are in agreement: formula is a very safe alternative to human milk. Other practitioners may break down this research differently than me, or your personal beliefs and risk assessments may not align. That's fine; follow the advice and information here that fits your circumstance, but know that I am writing from the perspective that safely prepared formula and breast milk are very comparable in growing healthy, happy babies and families.

HUMAN MILK

WHAT'S IN IT?

Fresh milk is a living tissue. Mind-blowing, right? It is designed to go directly from a body into a mouth. Just like any food, milk is made of three macronutrients—protein, fat, and sugar—and a bunch of extra vitamins and minerals. The ratio of these macronutrients in milk varies a lot species to species but is pretty stable in humans. The kind of fat and the amount of fat in our milk does vary a bit. It can vary from person to person or day to day.

The moment milk is expressed it starts digesting itself, activating immune factors, and changing. This is the most significant difference between breast milk and formula: formula does not contain live immunity. Scientific understanding of the gut biome and its relationship to immunology is still emerging. We know that breast milk "seeds" the infant gut in lots of important ways; we just don't know yet what an impact that has. Many other correlations can be drawn, but we don't actually understand how milk-based immunity works, so a lot of that is interesting but not worth hanging your hat on as causation. For instance, we know that vaccination for COVID-19 in pregnancy is protective for infants, and we know there are COVID-19 antibodies in the milk of nursing parents with COVID infections, but for now we don't actually know if or how those antibodies in milk are protective. My big take away after years of study and reading a lot in the *Journal of Human Lactation*: breast milk is very, very cool, and formula is a very effective substitute. Both have risks and benefits. Because formula is based on breast milk, both formula and human milk contain roughly the same amounts of proteins, carbohydrates, fat, vitamins, and minerals.

HOW WE MAKE HUMAN MILK

Fresh milk is a combination of nutrients and bioactive factors that have a whole lot of different roles in our babies' bodies. Before it can do that, it must be made, and it is made in an *alveolus*, a.k.a. a "milk factory cell."

These little milk factories are clustered together like a bunch of grapes. Arteries surround each one, bringing blood flow to a circle of milk-making cells, called *lactocytes* or *mammary epithelial cells*. Inside this ring of cells is a *lumen*. You can think of the inside of the lumen as a balloon where the ingredients of milk making accumulates until milk synthesis is triggered. Some substances are small enough to pass through the spaces between these milk-making cells right into the lumen, some pass through the cells, and some are made in the cells.

Milk is mostly water (about 87.5 percent). The water for making milk is attracted a type of sugar called *lactose*, which is made from the glucose (another type of sugar) in your bloodstream and the galactose synthesized by mammary cells. This is a complex process involving a few different enzymes, but I won't make you go that deep into biology class. Just know that human milk is made on demand, and some substances easily get into it and others don't. While the energy to synthesize milk get stored up in the cells of a breast, the actual milk is made à la minute.

Next up are the fats: these either come directly from your diet or go from fat stores in milk-making cells into the lumen. Research led by nutrition scientist Maryanne Perrin has shown that a big difference between milk produced by one person or another is fat content and profile. She compared the diets of vegans, vegetarians, and omnivores and found differences in the unsaturated fats and transfats in their milk.[4] While the nerd in me is so fascinated by this, remember: different isn't better or worse. There doesn't appear to be any difference in health from babies who get different fat profiles. So there is no indication that you should be on a special diet while nursing.

Later in this chapter, you will learn how to read the back of a formula can, but in the ingredients list, you will notice the same dynamic as in breast milk: water, sugar, fat, protein, and then a whole long list of other important ingredients in very small amounts. Unlike in formula, in human milk, you would also find white blood cells, antibacterial components and other living immune factors, and a bunch of enzymes. I won't drag you too far into nerding out about these, but know that they are there, in varying amounts, and they are cool.

There is one nutrient concern in human milk: a conspicuously low amount of vitamin D. Vitamin D is very important for the proper function of the immune system and maintaining or developing bone density. Nature's assumption is that your baby will synthesize this vitamin from lots of time in the sun. For reasons involving shade, houses, and skin cancer, we no longer expect our babies or ourselves to get enough vitamin D from the sun. Instead, you should give your baby vitamin D drops in keeping with the recommendation of your child's doctor. You can also take larger amounts of vitamin D yourself, and it will translate into higher vitamin D quantities in your milk. Again, see your doctor for the appropriate dosages.

Now that the macronutrients are assembled, the vitamins, minerals, and immune factors cross the alveoli, and tada! Milk.

Once the milk is made, oxytocin stimulates cells that surround the alveoli, called *myoepithelial cells*, to contract, pushing milk out of your nipple like a tiny shower head.

WHAT GETS INTO OR AFFECTS MILK

Now that you understand how milk is made, it is easier to un gets into milk and what lifestyle changes are important to safely feed baby. When you are pregnant, your baby shares your bloodstream. For this reason, you have to be extra careful about what goes into your body. During nursing, however, it is slightly different, as most (but not all) substances get triple filtered before they reach your baby's bloodstream. Anything you ingest first gets filtered through your liver, then filtered again during milk synthesis, and then one more time when it goes through your baby's liver and into their bloodstream.

Your diet

In almost all cases, our bodies are so determined to feed our baby that it will take every nutrient you've got and put it in milk. If you don't get enough water or nutrients to refill the reserves in your body, you will start to feel pretty bad long before the quality or quantity of your milk changes much. I remember once pumping and forgetting to drink water in the NICU. When I told my midwife I was starting to see stars, she asked me if I had had any water that day. Oops. I was cruising toward full dehydration, but my body was still cranking out milk for my baby. Personally, I find this biology a little bit rude, but we are built to protect our babies. You should check in with your doctor if you suspect any deficiencies—for instance, vegan parents should consider B12 supplements to make sure they are passing enough of that vitamin on.

Research on organic food and breastfeeding also shows no meaningful difference in health outcomes. Some organic or fresh (and fresh frozen) foods may be higher in nutrition than processed foods, which may help you feel well.

Medication

I often hear from parents that they were told to pump and dump or stop nursing due to medication that wasn't actually incompatible with nursing. In reality, most prescription and over-the-counter drugs are safe. Drug companies do not spend the money and time to study these drugs in nursing people, and most doctors make decisions based on the manufacturer's label. If you are having surgery or taking a medication, have your doctor review the work of pharmacist and researcher Thomas Hale, who runs the LactMed lab in Texas. This lab is the leader in the field of medication and lactation. You can go to https://www.halesmeds.com and download his app, or recommend to your doctor that they do so, to get in-depth information on drug transfer into breast milk.

It is a very valid and reasonable choice to choose taking an incompatible medication over breastfeeding. Your baby needs a healthy parent more than they need breast milk.

Alcohol

The short version: "Casual use of alcohol (such as one glass of wine or beer per day) is unlikely to cause either short- or long-term problems in the nursing infant, especially if the mother waits 2 to 2.5 hours per drink before nursing, and does not appear to affect breastfeeding duration."[5]

Let's begin with the understanding that your milk alcohol level and your blood alcohol level are the same. There are also many factors that can impact your blood alcohol level, most notably the fact that you probably haven't had a drink in almost a year. So, an easy barometer to use is whether you would feel safe to drive.

Let's say your blood alcohol is .08 percent (the legal driving limit in most states). Your breast milk would now contain around the same amount of alcohol as some nonalcoholic beers. That is to say, your milk, which is a drink, has trace amounts of alcohol in it but not very much at all. Because of this, it is generally considered safe to nurse if you would feel comfortable driving. It is also fair to say that much beyond that limit, you probably aren't in great shape for parenting or driving and should have another caregiver step in. When your blood alcohol returns to zero, so does your milk. So, if you feel like your blood alcohol level is above a good nursing level, just wait an hour or two and you should be good to go, no need to "pump and dump." In fact, pumping and dumping has been shown to be ineffective.[6]

You can express milk while drunk if you need to do so to stay comfortable, but it will not clear alcohol from your breast milk. Very little breast milk is stored, it is made on demand. You do not need to pump and dump. You can just wait until you sober up a bit and nurse then.

If you are not comfortable with any amount of alcohol being in your milk, you can use the LactMed "Time to Zero" calculator to predict when your milk will be completely alcohol free.[7]

Alcohol has been shown to decrease milk production because it inhibits oxytocin.[8] If you are worried about low production, you may want to skip alcohol while you problem-solve.

Nicotine

While some nicotine can get into milk, the primary concern is second- and thirdhand smoke. If you smoke cigarettes, it's good to do so outside and away from your baby. Wash your hands and change clothes before feeding your baby.

THC

We still do not have good research on the impacts of THC—the psychoactive component in cannabis—on babies, mostly because it would be very unethical to expose babies to THC in order to study these effects. Instead, we rely on sound scientific logic and animal studies to conclude that cannabis is not safe while nursing. THC binds very well to fat molecules and is pretty bad for developing brains. Fat-bound chemicals also don't dissipate over time in the same way that other chemicals do (like ethanol in alcoholic drinks). This means they can stay in your bloodstream for days or weeks after, so there isn't a known safe amount of time to wait after ingesting THC. It's recommended that you avoid it all together until you are done nursing.

Cannabis has many medical uses, including the control of anxiety or PTSD, which are common in postpartum people. You should treat it like any other drug and review alternatives with your doctor that are safer while nursing or choose to wean and continue cannabis use.

Other drugs

In general, unregulated drugs are considered unsafe for nursing because of lack information about what may be in them. For instance, cocaine is very unsafe for babies. While it leaves your system within 24 hours, which would allow you to safely nurse after you are sober, we do not know what else is in it. There could be other unknown drugs that stay in your system and in the milk much longer. So, in general, unregulated drugs should be avoided completely while nursing or pumping.

Methadone: Methadone is considered safe if prescribed and monitored, and your medical team should be able to counsel you on using it while nursing.

Transdermal medications

Transdermal medications will have different indications for nursing/handling a baby. Since these are designed to go through the skin, you should be careful if the application site is somewhere that your baby touches often or that contacts their skin while feeding. For instance, testosterone can be applied topically and is safe for nursing. Testosterone molecules are too large to go into milk, but testosterone gel can go from your skin to your baby's system via their skin. If you are using a transdermal medication, talk to your provider about effective application sites that wont come in much contact with your baby.

Topical medications

These medications treat the skin. The most common ones you will come into contact with during this life phase are ointments for healing nipples. Most over the counter ointments are made of a variety of oils and are safe for your baby. Another great topical healing ointment is pasteurized honey. These medical honey ointments are anecdotally very effective, but you need to make sure they are pasteurized. The honey we eat can contain botulinum toxin (like in botox or the scary stuff in home canning), and is not safe for babies under one. Prescription nipple medications, like an antibacterial, antifungal, or steroid are also considered safe to nurse with, but you should speak with your pharmacist for specific recommendations.

Other vitamins

It is recommended that you stay on a prenatal multivitamin with iodine while nursing. This helps make sure you have enough vitamin stores to stay healthy, feel good, and have enough to pass on to your baby through your milk. Vitamin D is a great example of a vitamin that we don't tend to have enough of on our own. You can take a large dose yourself and your baby will receive it through your milk, or you can give them drops directly. Your doctor or baby's pediatrician should be able to help you calculate that dosage and chose a good prenatal vitamin.

Prebiotics and probiotics

Some people may want to supplement their baby by adding probiotics to their own diet. This may work; it may not. In reality, we don't yet understand enough about the transfer of probiotics and their function to know that this will work or which ones or how much. If your stomach is upset or you've had antibiotics, you may want to supplement your diet with a probiotic and trust that nature is on it. Manipulating your microbiome may impact your risk factors for mastitis. If you are using pre/ pro biopics to prevent mastitis look for ones with the following strains: *Limosilactobacillus fermentum* or *Ligilactobacillus salivarius*.

Check with your pediatrician, but if your baby seems to need some digesting help, you can offer a probiotic in addition to your milk and see if it helps.

IMMUNITY, INFECTION, AND MILK

Airborne viruses. Breast milk fans love to talk about the immune-boosting properties in milk. Truth be told, we know that human milk does have an impact on rates of some infections, but we don't fully understand how this occurs. This impact is also relatively small on an individual basis. What we do know is that we see lower rates of GI infections and eczema in breast-fed babies population wide.[9] Risk of infection on its own may not be a robust enough reason to nurse, but if you are already nursing, it's a good idea to nurse through any colds or viruses you or your baby may have.

Vaccination and milk. You should get vaccinated while you have a baby. From a disease transmission and public health standpoint, this is just good scientific sense. That being said, being vaccinated while nursing does not have a proven impact on a baby's immunity in the way vaccinations while pregnant do. We know that antibodies from vaccination do pass into milk. What we don't know is how those antibodies work in babies' bodies. Do those antibodies move through the digestive system and create immunity there? How much immunity is acquired? Best practice here is to stay up to date on vaccinations while pregnant and nursing to avoid getting sick yourself and spreading pathogens to your baby. I also recommend that you follow your pediatrician's vaccine schedule for your children.

Blood-borne pathogens. Some viruses pass through secretions. Unlike airborne viruses that spread through the air, these viruses spread through sex, blood exposure, or in rare cases, nursing or birth. Notably, viruses like HTLV, syphilis, HIV and hepatitis C and B can be transmitted via milk. Donors donating to milk banks are screened for viruses, and when sharing milk informally with peers, you should ask if they have tested positive for either of these viruses.

Herpes viruses pass through skin-to-skin contact. While rare, these viruses can appear on nipples and are dangerous to babies. If you notice any sores or breakouts on your chest, you should talk to your doctor immediately to rule out a HSV (herpes simplex virus) outbreak.

DONOR MILK AND WHERE IT COMES FROM

Another way that humans have fed our babies is by sharing milk with one another, known more commonly these days as *donor milk*. A long history of wet nursing both consensually and forced complicates this history. To mitigate these ethical dilemmas, our current milk-sharing system is mostly based on altruistic milk sharing. This happens through formal milk donation through milk banks and peer-to-peer milk donation from one parent's freezer to another.

The system of formal milk donation exists primarily in a medical context through a nonprofit organization called Human Milk Banking Association of North America (HMBANA). Now that we understand how lifesaving human milk can be for preemies, we have a system to guarantee them access to human milk regardless of their parents' ability or desire to produce it. This milk is distributed based on supply: first to the NICUs for medically fragile babies, then to healthy term babies who need supplementation in the first few days after birth, and then in times of abundance, the milk banks may sell milk or have it available for home use with a prescription. The cost and unpredictable supply chain make this an unsustainable solution for long-term supplementing, but formal milk banks are a great way to support medical milk management.

Milk donors are educated by HMBANA on safe milk collection practices and what status changes they should report during regular communication over the course of their donor period. They are screened and ruled out if they smoke, use unregulated drugs or take medication that is not safe for nursing, are at risk for CJD (commonly known as "mad cow disease"), and then they are tested for HIV, hepatitis B, C, HTLV, and syphilis.

Milk from these donors is then collected, tested again, pooled into large batches and pasteurized. Random samples are taken from these pooled batches and are tested again. This milk is then put in sterilized bottles and frozen.

There are still hypothetical risks to using donor milk, but they are very slim. It is not uncommon to be asked to sign a waiver for donor milk use in a hospital acknowledging that these small risks exist.

Milk banks ask that donors handle their milk more carefully than parents do when feeding their own healthy term babies, and because of the pasteurization, this milk is less able to fight its own bacteria and should be handled carefully once it's thawed. You would be receiving this milk from a medical provider who should give you recommendations on how to handle it safely.

A NOTE ON ANONYMITY OF DONORS AND POOLING

Close records are kept on every batch of donor milk and its safety and testing, but records are not released about *who* that milk came from. This information is only used for contamination/viral contact tracing. Milk banks cannot release information on donor identity to you, which can be a religious conflict for Muslims with a strict adherence to the Koran. If you have a religious conflict with using pooled milk but have a preemie who is at risk without it, you should talk to your medical team about the possibility of direct milk donation from a family member or community member.

Informal or peer-to-peer milk sharing

This kind of milk sharing is a broad spectrum that includes everyone from sisters offering one another milk to strangers from the internet driving cross-country to pick up coolers. Despite the occasional clickbait news story about milk purchased online and shipped warm, most milk sharing is actually very safe. Online and personal communities love helping each other by sharing their milk with one another.

A listing of available milk will look something like this:

I have about 118 oz of milk I'm looking to donate. My baby unfortunately can't drink my frozen stash because of a dairy and soy intolerance. Milk was expressed between 9/6–10/12.

Medications: I take prenatal, magnesium, and vitamin D supplements every day. I sometimes take Excedrin which is safe while breastfeeding.

I am located in ___________.

These boards about sharing and receiving milk are some of the most heartfelt places I have ever seen on the internet. They're a true home of mutual aid.

Some things to keep in mind when using shared milk

You should feel comfortable asking the same questions of a milk donor that you would ask a sexual partner: Do you have any exposures that put you at risk for HIV, hep B, or hep C? Are you taking any drugs incompatible with milk sharing?

It is not recommended to exchange money for milk outside of the context of a milk bank. While I feel strongly about the autonomy of people to do whatever they wish with their bodies, there is a concern that paying for milk incentivizes watering milk down or selling milk that ideally would go to that person's own baby.

It is customary to help a milk donor with supplies. Many milk donors will ask that you replenish their stash of milk-storage bags.

The riskiest part of milk sharing is transport. I recommend finding a milk donor within driving distance and getting frozen milk from their freezer into a cooler and then put directly into your freezer.

It is less common but possible to nurse another person's baby. In this instance the same questions should be asked as those you would ask a milk donor, as well as inquiring about any possible herpes virus outbreaks. A question you should also ask before anyone kisses your baby, incidentally.

FORMULA

The short version: for newborns choose a partially hydrolyzed formula that's easily available at your local grocery store.

When it comes to feeding babies, the FDA (Food and Drug Administration) doesn't mess around. The approvals and regulations for formula are closer to what we see with medications than with other foods. While formula companies are given more leeway with marketing claims and front-of-the-can labels than is probably good for families, the actual ingredients and nutrient ratios are tightly controlled. This means that, broadly speaking, with a typical baby, you can't go wrong. There also truly is not a "best formula." They are all slightly different to align with different budgets, preferences, and digestion needs. When you stare down the giant formula aisle, what you will see is a lot of bright-colored cans making a lot of claims about brains and guts and how close the contents are to human milk. While formula is very well regulated, these claims aren't. So, the first thing to do is turn the can around and look at the ingredients. You'll see something like this:

NONFAT MILK LACTOSE, VEGTABLE OILS, WHEY PROTEIN, AND LESS THAN 2% of . . .

The ingredients before the "less than 2%" are the ones that vary significantly from formula to formula. The ones after that vary, but in such small ways that they aren't worth too much investigation. Notice how, just like in human milk, the first few ingredients are: carbohydrates (sugar), fat, and protein. These three macronutrients can come from different sources in different ratios. They are all safe and healthy for babies, but some are easier to digest, more similar to human milk, or just plain agree better with your baby's system.

There is no one recommendation for "the best formula." You'll know if a formula works well for your family if it is within your budget, easy to get, and your baby has regular soft solid stools on it. If you notice constipation, diarrhea, bloating, or skin rashes, you may need to consider a more specialized formula or try switching a few times to find one that works better for your baby. In most circumstances, the need to switch comes down to the ratio of whey and casein, source of fat, or kind of sugar. This isn't something you can predict until your baby is born. You cannot know what works best with out little trial and error. There is a short explanation of what adjustments to formula can be made below, but this is something I get into in more depth on in "Troubleshooting" (page 146).

For now, you have to start somewhere. I recommend starting with a partially hydrolyzed formula (meaning the proteins are more broken down) and then after four months switching to a fuller-protein option. These are available in a range of: organic, generic, and slightly different ratios of the two main proteins in milk: whey and casein.

THROW OUT WHAT YOU THINK YOU KNOW ABOUT NUTRITION

Baby nutrition and adult nutrition are very different. Babies' bodies and brains are growing fast, and they need a lot of calories, and a lot of sugar, to do so. It should not alarm you how much sugar is in formula; that is a good thing and resembles the high sugar content of milk humans make. In the US, the most common alternative sugar source is corn syrup. This gives some people an immediate ick factor. Don't worry, it's still sugar, just fructose instead of lactose. Government farming subsidies make it less expensive than other plant-based sugars like brown rice syrup, but the end result of fructose is functionally the same.

A FEW EXTRA FORMULA TIPS

If your baby seems very uncomfortable, for example, is bloated, has skin rashes, constipation, or diarrhea, you may need to adjust formulas. Look at those first few ingredients on the can and try switching one variable at a time.

Switching proteins
Whey and casein are the major proteins in milk. Human milk has more whey in it than cow or goat milk, so some formulas add in extra whey to mimic this. This works great for some babies and is harder to digest for others. Your baby may be more comfortable with a formula with more casein in it.

Switching sugars
Lactose is very easy for babies to transform into energy, though other sugars are safe and good alternatives. Some babies don't make enough lactase (the enzyme that helps digest lactose) and will be sensitive to lactose formulas. If your baby has an upset stomach, you can slowly switch to one with less lactose and see if it is a better fit.

Switching fats
Needing a change in the fat used in formula is extremely rare. If changing the protein ratios and the sugar source doesn't help your baby digest comfortably, talk to your pediatrician.

You should also ignore marketing gimmicks like "plant-based." While kids and adults should get lots of vegetables in our diets, the formulas that come from other mammals are the closest to breast milk. Only use soy formula if you are vegan or if your doctor recommends it for your baby's specific health condition.

If you have WIC (food assistance for parents with Medicaid and their babies, or for babies in foster care) you will be issued the formula the state has a contract with. If it doesn't sit well with your baby, your pediatrician can write a prescription for something that is easier on your baby's digestion.

Avoid buying formula from international import stores or discount stores. There can be issues with recalled formulas being sold or relabeled outside of standard grocery stores. After your baby is six months, however, these are generally the best places to get avocados and mangos.

If your family takes a special interest in the environmental or social impacts of certain companies or ingredients, you can start with a formula that is more aligned with your values. Some families have political oppositions to Nestle, or environmental questions about palm oil, or they want organic products. You can do research and choose one that is right for your family; remember that these differences are political, not nutritional.

THE BASIC RECIPE OF FORMULA (ALL FDA-REGULATED FORMULA)

Skim cow's milk + fat (because the fat was removed from the cow's milk, usually replaced with vegetable oils to make it more similar to human milk) + extra minerals that are needed for human babies + extra vitamins needed for human babies + extra carbohydrates needed for human babies.

THE FRONT OF THE CAN

Remember: The marketing on the front of the can doesn't matter. Look at the back of the can. That being said, here is a breakdown of what some of these words from both the back and front of the can mean about farming, ingredients, and marketing:

Organic

Organic formulas are made using ingredients that meet the standards of USDA organic certification. That means the ingredients are grown and animals are raised without any of the chemicals on the list of prohibited substances. Chiefly, these are: pesticides, chemical fertilizers, and dyes. While some organic foods may contain variations in nutrition over conventional versions, formula has all of those nutrients very carefully measured and adjusted, so these variations are unlikely to make any health difference in formula. Most research on the subject has found lower levels of trace pesticides in the urine of people who eat mostly organic. We do not, however, have any good research on what that means and the causative effects of an organic diet.[10] Large-scale organic farming is better for the environment than large-scale nonorganic farming. If your family prefers organic for any of these reasons and can afford it, an organic formula may be a good fit for you. Start there, and if your baby cannot digest it well, you may need to shift between organic options or opt for a conventional option.

Non-GMO

This means that the ingredients in this can of formula have not been genetically modified. Most organic formulas are also non-GMO. The science on GMOs (genetically modified organisms) is fairly new, and we honestly don't know yet if they are good or bad.

Now with added . . .

You may see ingredients here like probiotic, prebiotic, DHA, lutine, lactoferrin, and milk fat global membrane. These ingredients make up a tiny percentage of what is in formula and a huge percentage of the marketing. None of these extras or additives have been shown to have a clear causation impact on long-term health or they would be required in all formulas. For these reasons, I would stick to reading the back of the can rather than the front of the can. If your doctor feels that your baby would benefit from any extras (like a probiotic or DHA, for instance) these things can be given separately as a supplement.

For supplementing

This label has very little meaning in practice. Many formulas are marketed for supplementing and are completely different from one another. Any formula can be used in combination with breast milk or on its own.

Gentle/for reflux/sensitive

These are marketing terms. If your baby is having an upset stomach or reflux (see page 206), then work with your pediatrician and use some of the tips on page 149 to try switching formula to something that may be easier for your baby to digest.

Partially hydrolyzed

In this kind of formula the proteins have been broken into smaller pieces to make them easier to digest. This also can reduce the reaction a baby has to a protein by making it smaller. If your family has a history of dairy sensitivity, this may be a good option.

Hypoallergenic (fully hydrolyzed)

In a hypoallergenic or elemental formula, the proteins are broken all the way down until a baby's immune system no longer recognizes them. This formula is expensive and, to be honest, stinky, so it is really only for babies with true allergies.

A2 MILK–BASED FORMULA

Cows that produce A2 proteins instead of A1 proteins make a milk that may be easier for some people to digest. While this hasn't been studied in babies in a significant way, there are some studies in adults and children that show that some people digest A2 milk more quickly and easily. If your baby isn't allergic to cow's milk but seems to be constipated or having an uncomfortable time digesting formula, an A2 formula may be worth considering. Remember that this is just one protein in one ingredient; different A2 formulas can be very different in their makeup overall, so look at the whole picture when choosing a formula for your baby's digestion.

GOAT MILK FORMULA

Goat's milk protein is very similar to that of cow's milk. So, while it is a possible alternative to cow's milk formula, it isn't a good option for babies with allergies to cow's milk. It is slightly easier to digest because the proteins are smaller and the milk forms softer curds. They also do not make A1 protein. So, goat milk formula may be similar for digestion to A2 cow's milk formula. Goat milk–based formulas have been available in other parts of the world for a long time. Recently, due to the formula shortage in 2022, the FDA has approved the use of and importation of more goat milk–based options.

GRASS MILK FORMULA

Cows that eat a grass diet have a different fat composition than cows who eat a diet with grains in it. This is similar to the way we see changes in parental milk fat depending on diet. Some people find that they digest grass-fed milk better. While less likely to impact digestion than protein (as with A2), grass fed may be a better fit if you are seeing troubled digestion in your baby. That being said, always look at the back of the can. If milk is from grass-fed cows but the formula is made with skim milk, there will be no dietary difference than non-grass-fed formula, because the difference (fat) was filtered out. Some people also just want milk from happier, healthier cows, in which case, go for it.

EUROPEAN FORMULA: WHAT TO KNOW

If you have the means and the will, you may find yourself leaning toward importing a European formula. European formulas are regulated by different bodies (Europe's versions of the FDA), and these bodies have different standards. There was once a time when some of these characteristics could only be found in European formula, but as their popularity has grown, American formula companies have started to make options that are very similar to what you might import from Europe. The big takeaway with European formula is that their overall standard is higher, so there is less of a range in the sourcing of ingredients, but similar formula characteristics can be found in US formulas.

Things to consider if you choose a European formula

The most important things to consider if you are considering a European formula are supply chain and storage. The popularity of this option has led to many "drop shippers" and redistributors that import European formula and store it in unregulated ways. There are also larger official distributors that are more transparent about their shipping practices. These are questions you should ask when looking into a retailer. Global demand for these formulas can make the supply chain unstable. You should source a similar US formula as backup if these supply-chain issues come into play.

Biodynamics/organic/pesticides

All European formulas are required to be what in the US is classified as organic. These biodynamic farming practices are better for the planet and have tighter surveillance of pesticides that come anywhere near your baby's formula. If this is important to you, you should source a US formula that is organic.

Less iron

European certifying bodies have a different interpretation of the iron needs of babies than the FDA. Therefore, they supplement their formula with less iron. European formula is also staged, meaning there are two blends that are appropriate for different age ranges. These stages have different iron values. If you have concerns about your baby getting too much iron, you should discuss this with your child's pediatrician.

DHA is required

While most US formulas have DHA in them, it is not required. European oversight requires it. It is fairly easy to locate a US formula that does contain DHA.

More soy-free options

A lot of US formulas contain soy somewhere in their ingredients. If there is a soy allergy or sensitivity in your family, you should talk to your child's pediatrician about good soy-free options, which may include importing a European formula.

Stages

European formula is designed in two stages: one for before six months and one for after six months. You should make sure you are buying the appropriate stage for your baby.

Country-to-country differences

The certifying bodies for different European countries are different. Some brands manufacture their formula for different countries and make it slightly differently for each country. Make sure that you are certifying the back-of-the-can ingredients you want and that you are always getting the same country's blend.

"European-style" formula

Organic, soy-free formula with DHA is going to be very close to a European formula. Some companies are even marketing themselves as "European-style." I encourage you to treat this just like any other formula and look at the back of the can to decide based on ingredients.

Different mixing ratios

Mixing the right formula ratio is extremely important. Imported formulas may have a different water-to-powder ratio. Be sure to read the can. The obvious concern here is that if the can isn't in a language you speak, you will have a problem.

Approximating European formula yourself

If you want to approximate European standards without having to deal with the precariousness of having your formula shipped to you try this: Start with an organic, partially hydrolized formula with added DHA, then after four to six months, move to an organic formula with DHA and a more whole protein.

SOY FORMULA

Soy formula (sometimes marketed as "plant-based" formula) follows the same recipe as cow's milk formula in its macronutrients, but because it doesn't come from a mammal, we have to add more of everything and process it more to get it closer to human milk. That means that soy formula is more processed than cow's milk formula and is not preferred. Vegans who cannot produce their own milk or do not want to use donor milk may find this their only suitable option, despite the fact that it is not completely vegan.

What about estrogen? There is no estrogen in soy, but it does have a component that estrogen receptors can be tricked into thinking is estrogen. There are some studies on this, but in all honesty, we just don't know if this has any effect on health and development.

Soy formula is never appropriate for premature babies because it does not contain enough absorbable minerals. It is only recommended for babies who have a (rare) genetic inability to break down lactose. This is very different from a lactose sensitivity or dairy allergy, which can be accommodated with other recommendations.

TODDLER FORMULA

These are formulas that, in order to work around the tight FDA controls for infant formula, are labelled for toddlers, for whom the regulations are much less strict. This allows companies to use ingredients like pea protein instead of soy, which hasn't been studied long enough for FDA approval. It also means that while they may meet the nutritional criteria for infants, you do not know that as a baseline. I don't recommend using toddler formula for your infant under six months. If you are doing some supplementing but mostly nursing after six months and consider formula a complementary food, you can check with your pediatrician about this option. As for formulas for toddlers, there is no nutritional need for a toddler formula. Toddlers can safely drink cow's milk or water and get all their nutrients from food.

PREMIXED VS. STERILE

Liquid formula comes in two forms: small bottles of sterile formula and premixed formula. These are much more expensive than powder you mix yourself, but the convenience of premixed is worth it for some families.

ANDY'S STORY

When they planned to have kids, Andy worried that his kids would be so genetically similar to his partner and sperm donor that he wouldn't be able to joke with them. "What if they were these smart introverted kids, and I had no one to joke around with?" As fate would turn out, Margot's eggs weren't usable and so Andy used his. In 2017, after much conversation and hope and trying, they conceived J.D. using Andy's egg and the sperm of a very smart introvert via reciprocal IVF.

Like a lot of parents, Andy struggled to find himself in his new role. "J.D. was so attached to Margot. He nursed around the clock." Margot was very clear in her desire to carry and nurse a baby. "When someone loves what they are doing and do it well, we let them do it and get out of the way."

For Andy there was another layer to the story. When J.D. was born, Andy wasn't out as trans yet. Being disconnected from himself made it hard to connect with his kid.

Things were different when the twins were born. Andy and Margot again did reciprocal IVF, and Andy had top surgery. He was starting to find his footing in himself, not just as a parent, but as a dad.

Remmy took to nursing immediately but had no interest in bottles, whereas Franny didn't want to nurse. They changed the plan. Margot went to work with Remmy strapped to her chest, nursing in a carrier, and Andy stayed home with J.D. and Franny and fed Franny bottles. Yes, they formula-fed one twin and breast-fed the other. As it turns out both babies had tongue ties that went unchecked due to the pandemic. The ties impacted how they ate differently and so they needed different things.

When Remmy and Franny got their first illnesses, it was a bad case of RSV that hit them identically despite having been fed different first foods. These days they are both happy, healthy, securely attached kids.

Sterile and premixed are not the same. Premixed formula is not sterile, but neither is any home-mixed formula, or breast milk for that matter, so it's perfectly fine for most babies. If your baby is very preterm, immunocompromised, or tube-fed, your doctor may recommend a sterile formula.

PREEMIE FORMULA

Premature babies have entirely different guts and dietary needs than their term counterparts. A lot of research has gone into this topic to make specific preemie formulas. Feeding preemies is more complex than feeding term babies, and so your baby's neonatologist and pediatrician will give a lot of guidance on what to use.

If your baby was late preterm (thirty-four weeks and older) your doctor may decide that they do not need specialized preemie formula. In that case, you will want to look for a low-lactose formula. Babies do not make enough of the enzyme lactase until they get closer to forty weeks, so a formula with other sugars may be a better fit until forty weeks, when you can switch gradually, if you'd like.

CHAPTER 5
NURSING

CHESTS AND BREASTS

Now that you know about what to feed a baby, we can delve into how to feed a baby. If you want to feed a baby with your body, understanding it is paramount. This means we are going to need to learn some anatomy. What a strange thing to have an organ system that jumps into action, requires hands-on maintenance, and is in a lot of ways completely new to you. I want you to be in control of your body, your choices, and your health. This is the starting place of nursing a baby, and it begins with understanding your own body.

SHAPES AND SIZES

This is a breast.

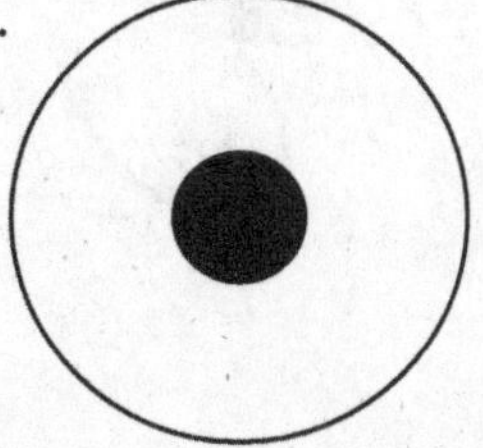

Just kidding, that is obviously not a breast. Breasts are not circular or symmetrical. Breasts are complicated. They are part of our culture and our self-esteem. They are part of our sex lives. Then suddenly, they change purpose and become about feeding a person.

Breasts and chests are diverse. Some have more glandular tissue; some have more fat tissue. Some people have everted nipples that stick out; some have flat nipples. Most people haven't spent a lot of time understanding these functional aspects of their chest. The goal of this section is to help you to understand your own body and become an authority on it. The idea that small breasts must produce less milk and that large breasts produce more milk is completely false. It is true, however, that breast history and shape can give us some insight into that breast's ability to produce milk. It's just not as simple as big versus small.

Do you see a breast in this typology that resembles your breasts or chest?

These guidelines apply to breasts after the first trimester of pregnancy.

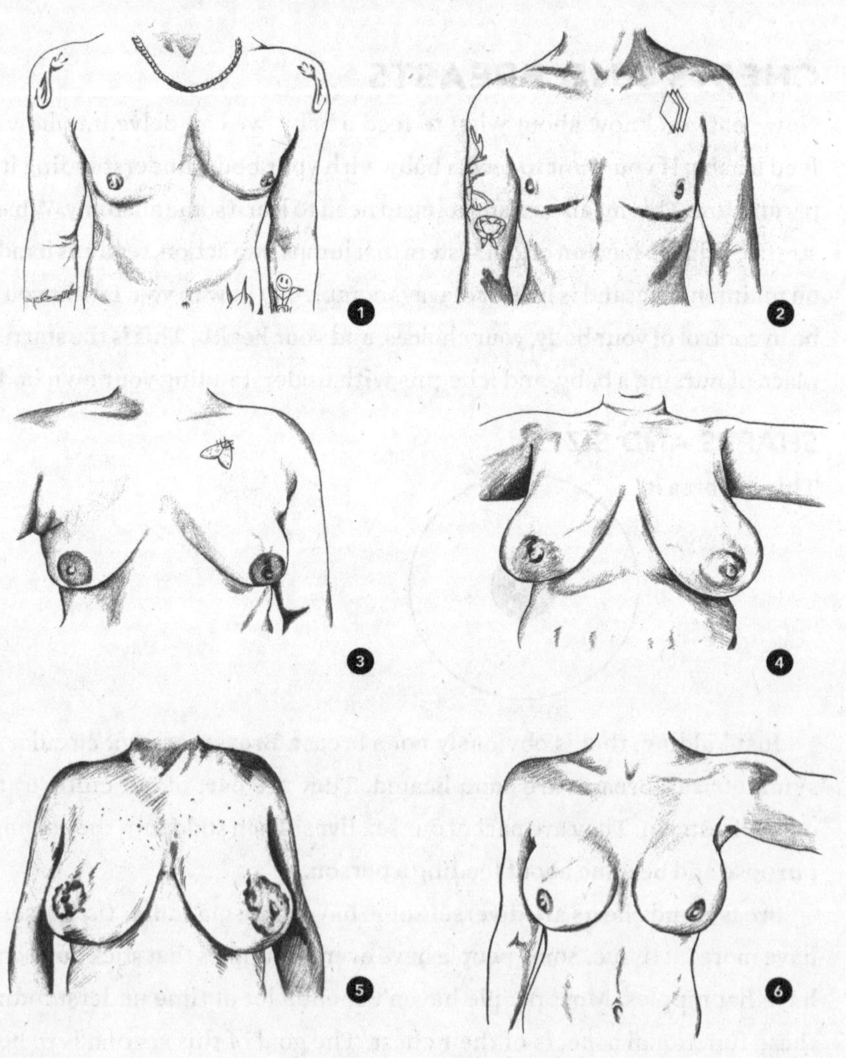

Our milk-making gland tissue changes a lot during pregnancy, so you may find yourself in a completely different place than where you started.

Not all breasts are represented here, but look for the best approximation or draw your own.

Asymmetrical breasts

First of all, your two breasts may be very different. When you are looking at these types, both may fall into one style or they may fall into two styles. They are, however, different from one another and each has a different nipple shape. Asymmetrical breasts or nipples might mean that you use different tools on each side, or that you or your baby may prefer one side to the other.

Small breasts (1)

Small breasts still grow during pregnancy. Generally they feel tight or full during pregnancy as breast growth fills up the available space. It is a misconception that small breasts produce less milk than large breasts. What matters are the hormones and milk-making tissue, not size.

Top surgery/mastectomy (2)

Surgically flat chests produce little to no milk because the lactation tissue has been removed. If you've had a complete mastectomy, then all of the breast tissue has been removed and you will not have breast-tissue growth in pregnancy. If you had top surgery for gender-affirming or aesthetic reasons, the surgery doesn't remove all of the breast tissue, and it is common to have some regrowth during pregnancy that may produce some milk. In either case, nursing is still possible, if desired, using a supplementary nursing system (page 269).

Tubular breasts (3)

Milk-making tissue feels pretty firm. If you feel around your chest and do not find much firm tissue, or if you have tubular shaped or wide spaced breasts, you may have less glandular tissue than you would need to feed a baby. This is often caused by a thyroid issue or medical or emotional complication during puberty. This style of breast is very common in people with PCOS. This is a risk factor for low production. If this is your breast type or you have a known thyroid condition, it is worth checking in with a lactation consultant to make a plan for if you don't make enough milk. This could be using a supplementary nursing system, supplementing with bottles, using formula and donor milk, etc. Understanding your risk factors for low production can help you start to make peace with it and empower you to adjust your expectations before you are sleep deprived.

Large or long breasts (4)

Large breasts have space for lactation tissue to grow during pregnancy and may change more in texture than size. Some have softer fat throughout or feel very full of firmer glandular tissue. Large breasts tend to be very heavy as glandular tissue multiplies and many find structured bras more comfortable. You may be glad to hear that the concept of underwires creating plugged ducts is a myth, and I recommend finding bras that continue to feel supportive in pregnancy and nursing but that fit well and do not block circulation. You may even find that you want a specific sleep bra. A few brands to try are: Kindred Bravely, Cake, and some good store brands at Walmart or Target.

A longer breast shape doesn't have any bearing on a person's ability to nurse. It may impact the positions you find comfortable to nurse in (page 107) and what bras you find comfortable.

Reduced breasts (5)

There are different styles of breast reduction surgery, but in general some of the duct tissue is removed and the nerves that are all around the breast are interrupted. You may also find that your breast tissue regrows somewhat during pregnancy. Some people who have had a reduction may be able to make a full supply of milk; some cannot. There is a huge range of surgical techniques and reasons for having reductions, so mileage will vary. You can use tools like pumping and galactagogues to maximize milk-making potential, or you might find that supplementing with donor milk or formula is necessary. This can be done either with a bottle or a supplementary nursing system (page 269).

Augmented breasts (6)

If you've had breast augmentation surgery, think about what your breasts looked like before surgery. If your breasts were one of the types that are at risk for low milk production, then that is a risk factor worth keeping an eye on. If your breasts were typical, then it is likely you will not have problems with milk production, though you may have some struggles with uncomfortable fullness and/or engorgement. It will also be more difficult to tell when your breasts are full or drained feeling, so you will want to pay closer attention to your baby's fullness cues and weight gain. I recommend paying particularly close attention to the portion of this book about engorgement and lymphatic drainage.

AREOLAS AND NIPPLES

Areolas are the darker ring of skin around the nipple. They vary in size from barely extending from the nipple to covering most of a breast. I've had many patients over the years describe themselves as having large nipples (usually a statement about themselves they have been carrying around since high school), when in reality, they have large areolas. Areolas darken in pregnancy to help babies find the breast and latch.

Areolas are also home to the occasional hair and to the Montgomery glands, little bumps on the areola that secrete a very convenient antimicrobial lubricant to keep your nipples from being infected or chapped, as well as a pheromonal smell that attracts babies to you. In sleep studies, anthropologist James McKenna found that breast-fed babies move very little in their sleep. They oriented themselves toward this smell and therefore stayed facing their nursing parent's chest through the night. Please respect the Montgomery glands and do not poke or pick at them. If one becomes irritated, talk to your doctor, but generally, it's best to leave it alone. As for the occasional hair, it shouldn't be a problem. Pluck them, don't pluck them: that's your business.

Nipples are about as varied as people themselves, but they do fall into three general categories: everted, flat, or inverted. That means that when your nipples are stimulated by cold or touch, it either firms up pointing out,

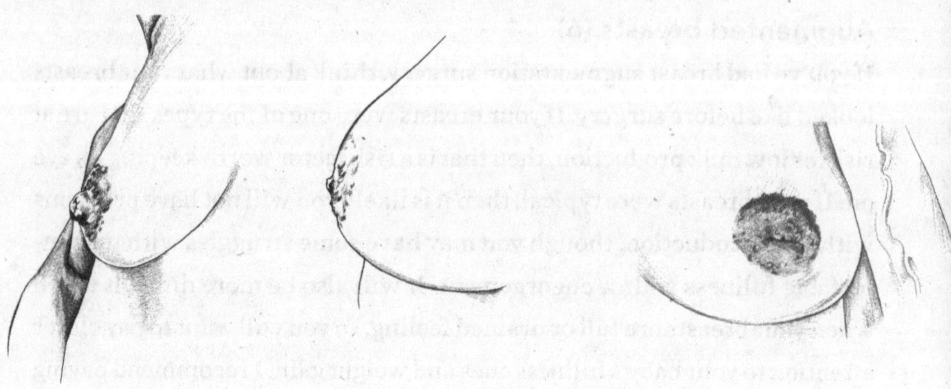

stays flat to your breast or firms up pointing in. When we get into latching in the next chapter, you will notice how far back in a baby's mouth a nipple needs to be to engage a suck (short version: it's like eating a taco, not drinking from a straw). Everted nipples are easier to elicit a suck with. It is not impossible, but is harder with flat or inverted nipples. Nipples can become flat when breasts are engorged, or evert over time with nursing and pumping. Nipple shields can help create a firm, everted nipple that helps a baby latch on (for more on this, see page 106). If you have flat or inverted nipples there is no need to rush out and get a shield; they will have them at your birthing place or the lactation consultant's office, where they will fit you for one if you need it. It is also not uncommon to have different nipple styles on each side, just to keep things interesting.

At the tip of your nipple you will find somewhere between 5 and 20 tiny outlets. These little pores at the end of each duct are where the milk comes out. If you want to visualize it, think of a shower head, not a faucet. This is fairly irrelevant when nursing, as all outlets are contained in your baby's mouth, but is delightful when discovering how to spray your partner in the face when they are annoying you.

Now that you have looked at and felt your breasts, let's take a look under the hood. Breasts are complex organs. They are full of glands, nerves, lymph nodes, and lots of blood flow. Think of this as a busy highway interchange: there's a lot going on, so sometimes traffic jams (plugged ducts) arise and things can go wrong (infections, bruises, swelling).

As you read this part, touch your chest and see if you can follow along. Feeling your chest is essential for lifelong health. You know this, but we could all do with a reminder. The more you know about what is normal for you, the better you can tell when something is abnormal or when you are getting ready to enter a new normal. Chests change a lot during pregnancy and over the span of nursing. A continued awareness of your body will help you notice new changes as you go. As you continue through this book, you will learn a hands-on approach to breasts. I hope this becomes part of your approach to routine health and gratitude for your body.

LAYERS OF THE BREAST

Nerves

Pain is common in nursing because, well, all these freaking nerves! The nerves extend throughout your breast, gathering at the nipple and communicating back and forth. This is why nipples are so sensitive. They communicate a lot about your baby back to your body and brain, including how frequently your baby eats or when to begin synthesizing milk and "let down" when milk starts flowing.

If you have pain, these nerves are communicating with you through that pain. It may be because your baby has an incorrect latch, and they are telling you to get help. (For help with latching, see the next section.)

Think of these nerves like a little lightning storm. When pain is bad, it will reverberate back and forth through the breast and out to the nipple. In some particularly bad cases, this can last long after nursing. I cannot overstate this: This. Is. Communication. Your body is trying to tell you something. Pain is common, but it is a sign that you need help. For the particularly stoic, toughing it out can cause lasting damage to these nerves. It is much better to address this pain than to tough it out and hope it gets better.

Blood flow

The next system working hard in the breast is the circulatory system. You may have noticed big bulging veins start to appear on your breasts in pregnancy or after milk transition. Milk is synthesized in the breasts on demand. That means that the water and nutrients to make milk come into your breast tissue through arteries, which act like highways.

Lymphatic fluid

Your lymphatic system is like the gutters of your body. Lymphatic vessels carry fluid around your body and moves excess fluid out of the way. Your armpits and clavicle are major junctures for your lymphatic system. This is also a big part of your immune system: when your body is fighting an infection, you often can feel swelling of the lymph nodes. When you are carrying excess fluid from birth or pregnancy, it will collect in the breasts, making them overly swollen. Your breasts are extremities. Like your hands and feet, they hang away from the body, so extra fluid tends to get stuck in them. Your lymphatic system is in charge of moving this fluid away and processing it, but as blood flow to your chest increases and ducts swell as they "turn on," it can cause an uncomfortable traffic jam. This is called *engorgement*, and it is very common in the first few days after a baby is born, but it can be recurrent for some people depending on their anatomy. You can find massage techniques to help this process along on page 162.

Glandular tissue

Glandular tissue feels like big lumpy bunches inside of a lactating breast. It pulls nutrients and water from those big blood vessels and passes them into the milk-making cells to be converted into milk. This tissue is clustered into little bunches like grapes called *lobules*, and those lobules are clustered into bigger bunches called *lobes*. The bigger bunches all branch together into ducts, which leave the breast through five to twenty outlets at the tip of the nipple. When speaking with breast surgeon and IBCLC Dr. Katrina Michell, she described

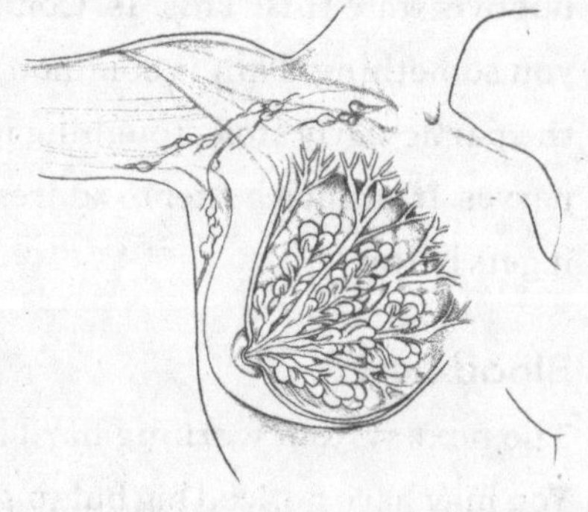

bunches of gland tissue as so tightly bundled and microscopic that you cannot actually see or feel them. You may feel swelling or inflammation in this tissue, but the actual glands are microscopic. Glands are sensitive and very different from muscles. For this reason, you should treat them gently and respectfully, like any other gland in your body. Think of any breast massage you do in terms of: Would I touch a cat like this? Soft touch is going to increase warmth, encourage oxytocin, and engage your lymphatic system, whereas rough touch can cause bruising and damage.

Ducts

Milk ducts connect the lobes of gland tissue to the nipple. They carry and eject the milk you make. These ducts are very small and fine, which means that fat can occasionally build up along them and create a clog. While they branch together into a larger duct right near the nipple, the ducts throughout the breast are microscopically small. This is why you cannot force a clog out of a duct using your fingers. For more on how to clear a clogged duct, see page 164.

Fat

Surrounding the glands is fat tissue, a.k.a. *adipose tissue*, which gives the whole system a little bit of room to expand and contract when full or drained. You may be able to feel the softer areas of fat surrounding the firmer areas of gland tissue in your breasts.

Now that you have all the information, it is time to literally take matters into your own hands. Look in the mirror; do a self-assessment.

- What type of chest do I have?
- Have I had surgery on my chest?
- Do I have everted, flat, or inverted nipples?
- Has my chest changed since getting pregnant/giving birth?
- Do I feel firm glands all the way around my breasts?
- Are my breasts different sizes?

I know this kind of self-reflection on our bodies can feel challenging, but knowledge is power. You are about to USE this system in a whole new way, and you deserve to be in charge of how you use it. You get to be in control of your health, your feeding choices, choosing your providers. You don't have control over everything in reproduction, but you do have control over knowing your body and using it how you choose.

HOW TO NURSE A BABY

If your baby hasn't arrived yet, the volume of information in this chapter might be a little overwhelming, but rest assured it'll be right here waiting when you need it. While a lot of this technique is fairly unimaginable right now, having it tucked into the back of your brain will serve you later. If you have arrived here in a moment of desperation, latching an uncooperative baby: hang in there; try these techniques; it'll get better.

BABY MOUTH ANATOMY

Now you've explored your own chest anatomy, join me in a little exploration of your mouth to understand your baby's mouth, which will help you understand exactly how the baby will latch on to a breast or bottle.

First touch under your jaw, between your chin and neck. That soft bit is the underside of your tongue. Feel how it connects to your throat and neck muscles? The tongue is part of a huge group of muscles connected to your jaw to help you breathe, eat food, and talk.

Now run your tongue along the roof of your mouth and feel your palate. Is it flat? Vaulted? Can you feel where your palate goes from feeling hard to soft allll the way at the back?

Now swallow. Feel how your throat coordinates your swallow so you swallow saliva and not air. Turn your head all the way to one side and swallow. Look up at the ceilings and swallow. Look straight ahead and swallow. See how the angle of the muscles in your neck impacts how you swallow. Being familiar with this will help you understand latch.

LATCHING

Latch—or as one of my mentors, Dr. Allison Stuebe, calls it, "the oral-boobular interface"—is the way that a baby's mouth aligns with a nursing parent's chest to transfer milk effectively and painlessly. It's another word for the shape a baby's mouth makes around a bottle or breast. It looks like this:

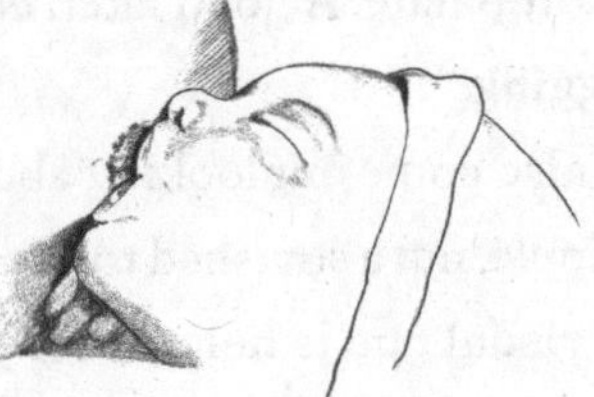

In order to draw milk into the mouth, a baby has to make a seal. This is done by *flanging*, or flaring big fishy lips out and drawing the tongue over the gums with the mouth open. The tongue makes a U-shape and touches the bottom lip making a nice big circle in contact with whatever kind of nipple a baby is eating from.

This seal creates the vacuum that draws milk into the mouth. Think about it like a suction cup: The baby makes a seal and then drops down their jaw making the suction pull and draw milk forward. This seal and vacuum are why the latch is so important.

The goal is the baby's gums and tongue are past the nipple, a.k.a. the area of the breast where all the nerves are, and are safely back on the breast where you have less sensation. This means that the compression of the baby's mouth happens up by the ducts and the suction comes not from compressing the nipple, but from a vacuum created in the back of a baby's mouth when they move their jaw up and down.

A little checklist for your latch:

- ☐ A big mouth full of breast tissue: like a taco, not a straw
- ☐ An active baby (though their eyes may be closed)
- ☐ Rolled up nice and close to you so their tummy is touching you

- ☐ You are seated comfortably, not hunched over your baby
- ☐ It feels like tugging, not pinching, not rubbing, not scraping.

If you are struggling to achieve these things: GET HELP!

To recap: a latch is like eating a taco, not drinking out of a straw. Your baby's mouth should be full of breast tissue with your nipple touching the back of their mouth at the soft palate. A good latch equals a deep, comfortable latch that feels like tugging.

Your nipple should also come out looking about the same shape it goes in—like a nice round nipple, not a smashed tube of lipstick with a line down the middle of it. This visual cue is helpful for people whose nerves fire atypically, and is a good quality check for anyone latching.

A NOTE ON MULTIPLES

I go into more detail about nursing multiples in the "Special Circumstances" section (page 263), but for now, know that when your babies are born (or if they are too little to eat just yet, as multiples are more likely to spend some time in NICU, when they are ready for oral feeds), you will start by feeding one baby at a time. This allows you to figure out what side they nurse best on and who needs more time or support to latch.

THE LATCHING "SMASH"

The best way to get a deep latch is to "smoosh" a big open baby mouth onto a breast like you are jumping into double Dutch or running into closing elevator doors. Again, think of taking a big (toothless) chomp out of a taco, not nibbling your way on. With a taco, all the good stuff will fall out, and with nursing, it'll hurt like a mother.

You can lead the smash, or your baby can. Most people prefer to do the parent-led smash in the early days because it gives you the most control, but I recommend trying both. There is no wrong way to latch a baby. If it works for you and you are both comfortable, I'm happy.

Baby-led smash

Note: Often not for people recovering from cesarean birth. Return to this when your incision is healed and leaning back is comfortable.

Babies have all kinds of reflexes that help them latch. Best yet, they look hilarious doing it. Letting your baby latch themselves can feel scary and out of control, but I invite you to try it with curiosity. In many cases, your baby is much better at latching than you, and this approach may unlock pain-free nursing. Lean back as far as you comfortably can (between totally flat on your back and about 70 degrees) and place your baby in the middle of your chest, below your nipples, tummy to tummy with you and with their little arms up like they are going to do baby push ups. Watch as they bob their way around, hunting for your nipple. You can redirect your baby, arrange or support your breast so it's easier to get to. You are allowed to help, but let them bob around and find it. Babies will often have some false starts and land on their fist or other breast tissue before using their sense of smell and rooting reflexes to finally push up into baby cobra and plop down right on your nipple, using gravity to hopefully get a pretty great latch. If it's an okay latch for you, but not a great one: use micromovements to improve it (page 104).

Parent-led smash

This is a better option if you have had a cesarean birth or have a disability where lying back is not comfortable.

Start in either football or cross-cradle position (page 108) and hold your baby with your arm along your baby's back, holding them confidently at the base of their head by the ears. This is your baby-wielding hand.

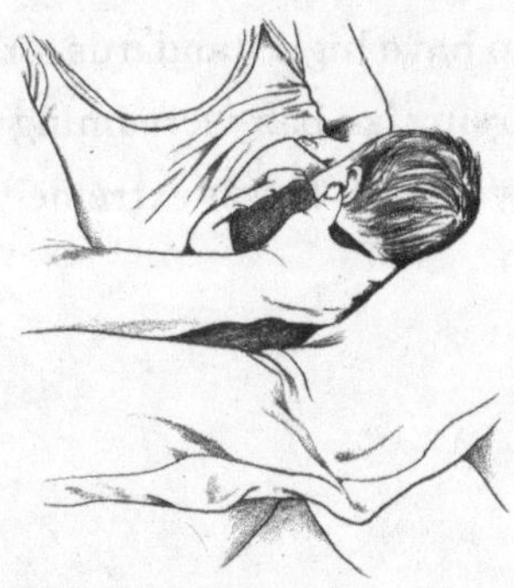

Use your other hand to make a taco with your breast.

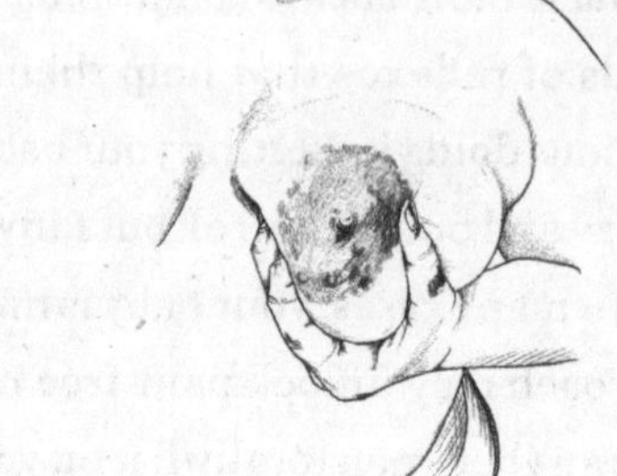

This is your chest-shaping hand. If you have small breasts, move your hand back as far as you can to allow for space for your baby to get that big mouthful. If you have large breasts you can use rolled up towels to support your breast and only need to taco the front four inches or so of your breast.

Using your chest-shaping hand, tickle the space between your baby's upper lip and nose with your nipple. This should trigger a reflex in your baby to open their mouth up. Pivoting their mouth up and over your nipple, smush that baby on.

This particular maneuver can be a bit like running through closing elevator doors or jumping into double Dutch. You will get the hang of it, but you might miss sometimes. If you miss the window, your baby may try to suck their way onto your nipple or be only latched to your nipple and not your breast. This will cause damage, which can cause pain. It can be so frustrating when getting a good latch is a screaming chaotic affair, but hang in there and try to have high standards. (Yes, you've been warned: A great deal of early nursing is a baby screaming directly into your breast while you try to collect yourself. This is extremely frustrating, but you can and will get through it.)

WHAT SHOULD LATCHING FEEL LIKE?

A good latch feels like tugging. It can feel intense, but it should not feel like pinching, rubbing, burning, or chomping. If even a deep latch feels like this, something is going on anatomically, and you should call a lactation professional.

WHAT SHOULD LATCHING NOT FEEL LIKE?

If you have ever taken new shoes on vacation, walked all over the place and gotten a blister, you know how it feels to have to face putting those shoes back on. You do not want your breast to feel like "blister shoes."

This is why we do not settle for a painful latch. Suffering through a bad latch can cause damage to the tissue that is hard to heal and is then painful to nurse on even with a good latch. It is normal to have some pain while you are figuring things out, but the goal is to strive for a pain-free latch and not cause tissue damage while you find your way there. No, your nipples will not toughen up. They are made of very delicate, thin tissue similar to the tissue on your lips. This is not like playing the guitar; nipple damage does not heal into helpful or cool calluses.

WHAT DO I DO ABOUT A PAINFUL LATCH?

In the spirit of not causing damage to your nipples that will take time to heal, you should stop a bad latch in its tracks and try again. I consider a bad latch as anything that makes you clench in pain, let alone yelp and curl your toes.

HOW TO UNLATCH A BABY

The best way I can describe it is to "fishhook" them. Let go of your breast taco with your chest-supporting hand and push your pointer finger into the corner of your baby's mouth along the gums. Pop the suction while keeping your finger between your baby's gums as you pull them away with your baby-

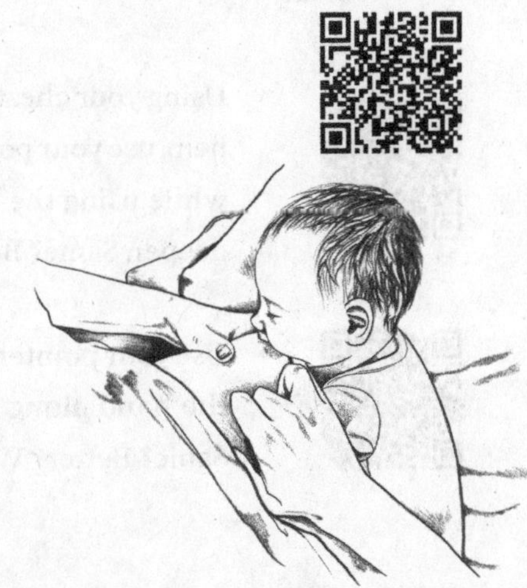

wielding hand. This will block your baby from chomping down as you pull your breast away, which is a natural reflex for babies. Take a deep breath and try again to smash your taco-ed breast into baby's mouth while it is as wide and possible.

Once you have smashed your baby into a latch using either the baby- or parent-led method, take a beat to take stock of this latch.

On a pain scale of 1–10, with 1 being "not painful at all" and 10 being "what is this untold torture," how would you rate this latch?

Early on, anything below a 5 is pretty normal. Some latches are kind of rubbing or uncomfortable but not outright painful. Use the techniques below to get that latch deeper and see if it can be improved.

Anything above a 5 is common but not okay. If your latches are above a 5, you should ask for help, unlatch, and try again. On page 281 you will find a feeding tracker where you can keep track of pain to see if it seems to be getting better, or it it is getting worse.

MICROMOVEMENT AND ADJUSTMENTS

These are small adjustments to try. Think of them like adding a pinch of salt or adjusting spices to your taste when you're cooking. Try them along with any intuitive small changes that come to you to see if you can get that all-important deep, effective, pain-free latch.

- Release your taco hand: Did that change the latch? Same? Better? Worse?

- Using your chest-supporting hand or asking a partner for help, use your pointer finger to pull your baby's chin down while using the baby-wielding hand to smoosh them on deeper. Same? Better? Worse?

- Use your pointer finger to flip up their top lip while using the hand along their back to smoosh them on deeper. Same? Better? Worse?

- Gently place a finger under their chin to support the tongue muscles. Just place it there. No need to push; it is just some extra support so baby can better coordinate a suck. Same? Better? Worse?

- Lean back so your baby is more on top of you, using gravity to pull their mouth more deeply onto your breast. Same? Better? Worse?

- Try moving your baby in small increments: slide their body lightly up. Slide them slightly down. Same? Better? Worse?

- Put another pillow under your baby so they are higher up, or take one out so they are slightly lower. Same? Better? Worse?

Is it common for it to hurt? Yes.
Should it hurt? No.

You and your baby are learning a high stakes, complicated partner dance. A certain amount of stepping on each other's toes is to be expected. Those latches will hurt. The goal is to recognize that the pain is trying to tell you something and to strive for better. On the whole, your latches should be trending toward getting better, but they will not simply get better as your baby grows or your skin toughens. The latch will improve as the two of you improve your technique. Again, consistent pain that doesn't improve with adjusting the latch is a sign of an anatomical problem and will not just "get better" on its own. A latch that makes you cry, yelp, or causes you to curl your toes in pain is cause for immediate concern and assistance. If you have access to a lactation professional, call one in immediately. In a pinch, an experienced friend who had a baby in the last year may be able to give you some help.

USING A NIPPLE SHIELD

A nipple shield is a thin piece of clear silicone that is shaped like a nipple. They are kind of like nursing training wheels for preemies or a mold for inverted or flat nipples. I find them to be frustratingly misnamed, as the word *shield* implies that they are intended to prevent abrasion or pain. They are not shields. They should not be used to shield from pain. They are nipple extenders.

They are an excellent tool for their intended purpose: assisting in shaping flat or inverted nipples or shaping a nipple for a learning preemie.

If you have flat or inverted nipples, there is absolutely no need to ever wean off the shield unless you want to. As babies grow, they often evert nipple tissue through nursing or get big and strong enough to latch comfortably onto breast tissue and suck without the reminder of the shield. The best way to do this is to start nursing with the shield and then remove it halfway through. If your baby latches well without it and you aren't in pain, you can gradually work toward an initial latch without it.

Shields can make nursing on the go trickier and add "one more thing" into the latch process (though some people do just keep them on between feeds for simplicity and a very striking look at parties).

If you don't have any of these specific circumstances, I recommend you avoid using a shield. They can be habit-forming for babies and may hide nipple damage by reducing pain but not resolving the underlying problem.

How to put on a shield

I recommend practicing this during times when your baby is not crying to be fed. It is a tricky motor skill, and it takes some focused learning.

- Dip the shield in water to help it stay in place on your nipple.
- Flip the shield partially inside out.
- Roll the shield over your nipple, flipping it back down so as much nipple is pulled into the shield as possible.

The shield should fit snugly but not feel tight. You may need to go up or down in size to get a good fit.

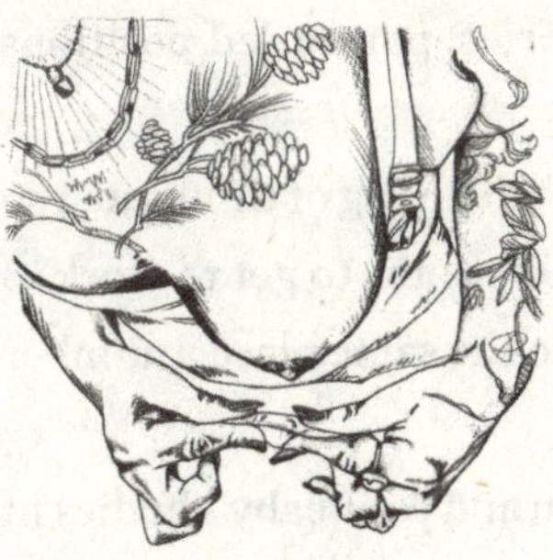

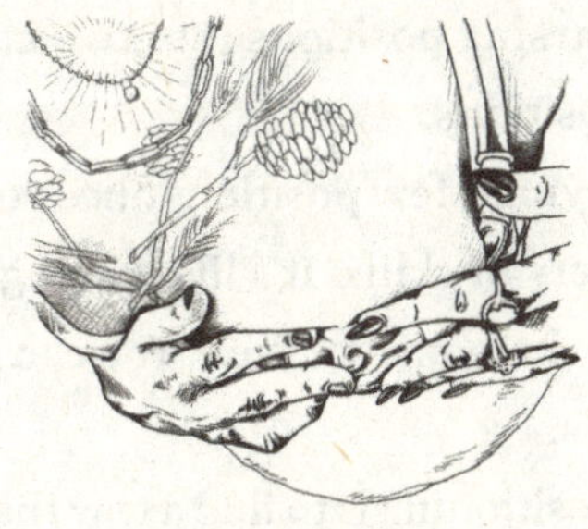

Sizing. Shields run from size 27 to 32. Ideally a shield will be fitted for you in your birthing place. If you know you have flat or inverted nipples, you should ask for a lactation consultant to come help you assess and size you. If you are pumping, you can use your flange size as an indicator.

Nipple shield tips

If you are home or don't mind a bit of silly looking protrusion, you can leave nipple shields on between feedings. This can save you a step when getting latched.

Wash your shields at least once per day in warm soapy water and have lots of them so that you have extras in a pinch. Keep one in your bag, one on your nightstand and one by the couch. They are the world's largest contact lens and get lost easily. You'll find it eventually, just go grab a spare. Keeping them in a container, like a retainer case, can make them easier to spot or grab out of your bag.

Avoid unusual shapes. Shields shaped like pacifiers, for example, can make latch and suck much worse. Avoid these unless directed by a lactation professional to use them intentionally.

FEEDING POSITIONS

There are infinite ways to hold your baby and nurse them. Over time, lactation professionals have broken down these possibilities into a few common holds to teach you. Most people find variations that work well for their bodies as they go along.

I separate nursing positions into two categories: parent-led positions and baby-led positions.

It is worth trying a few positions once you get the hang of things just so you have a variety of skills. It's like having a few routes to get to work in case one of them has construction. You can get to the same place a number of different ways.

The goal in positioning is to find a way that you and your baby's bodies fit together where you have a deep comfortable latch, your body is comfortable and supported, and your baby can manage milk flow well.

PARENT-LED POSITIONS

The classics: cross-cradle and football

These positions are nearly identical. To go from cross-cradle to football takes just a slide over, rather than a flip. If you are nursing a baby in football under your right arm, you can slide them along your body to be lined up with your left breast: et voilà—cross-cradle.

In cross-cradle, your arm is along your baby's back and supporting them behind the ears. Baby is propped up on your lap across your body in front of you. Their mouth is perpendicular to your body, and you are tummy to tummy.

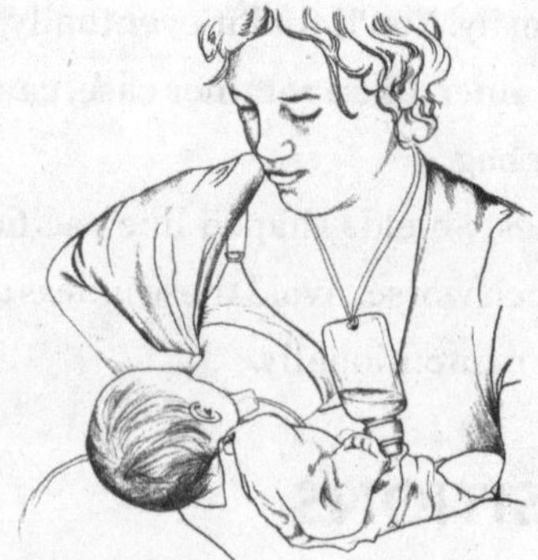

Football is exactly the same as cross-cradle, but shifted to where baby is tucked under your arm. I recommend building up vertical pillows behind your back to get set up for football, as babies have a "stepping reflex" and will kick away from a surface if it touches the bottom of their feet.

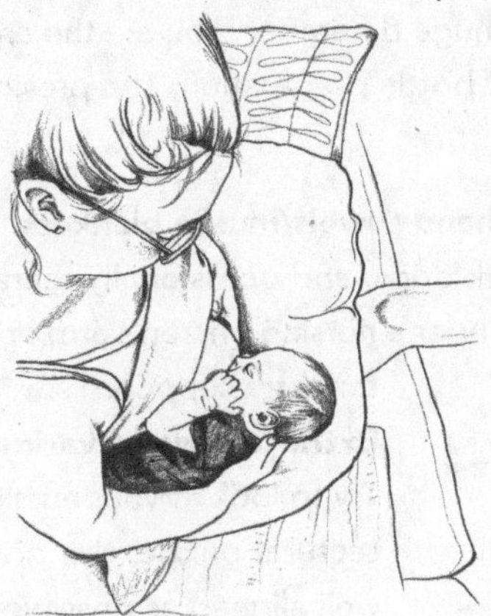

The Australian position

In this position your baby sits straddling your leg or a pillow (depending on y'all's heights in relationship to each other), facing you upright. Your baby's mouth is parallel to yours, so you will support your breast in a hamburger style. Just as with football or cross-cradle, you hold your baby's head at the base near the ears and have good control of how and when you latch. This position is great for mixing things up if you've had some nipple damage or for babies who don't like resting on their side. It is a little finicky with floppy babies, so it's okay if it feels awkward or uncomfortable; just try something else.

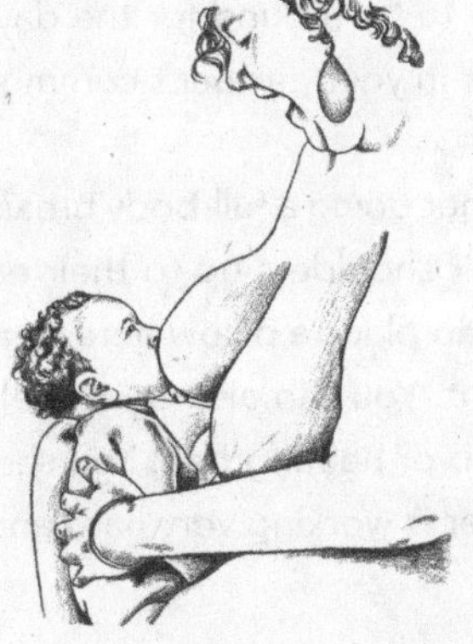

PARTNERS, CO-PARENTS, AND SUPPORT PEOPLE

You are essential here. You have free hands and a different perspective, so coming in for the assist in early days when babies are floppy and everyone is learning makes a huge difference. You are the architect of the feeding spot. The captain of bottle preparation. The president of spit-up cloths.

GETTING SET UP

A few burp cloths/hand towels/muslin blankets. These can be used to mop up spit-up, milk drips, and occasionally tears. They are also great to roll up and tuck under a nursing person's arm or behind a baby's back for extra support.

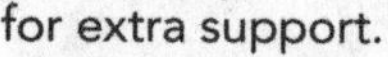

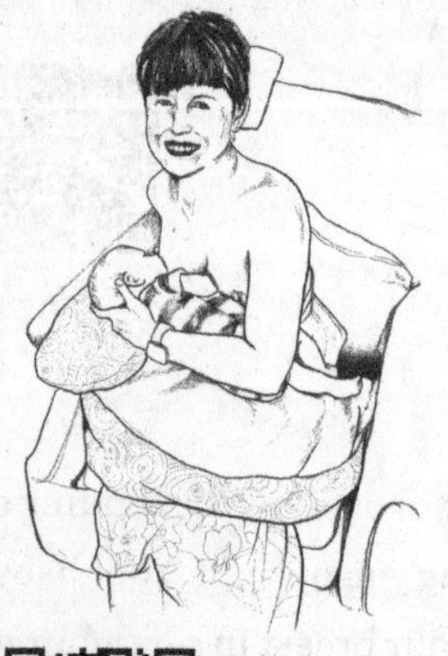

Extra pillows of various shapes and sizes. Try to look at your nursing dyad like an architectural puzzle: the goal is to have baby as well aligned as possible to the nipple with as little body effort as possible on the part of the nursing person. If they are hunching over baby, then baby isn't high up enough. Try stuffing pillows under whatever top nursing pillow baby is on. If baby is rolling away from the chest: roll up a cloth to line up behind baby.

Snacks. Nursing around the clock is hard work. Once the nursing parent is settled into a feeding, you can see if they are peckish and offer a bit of a granola bar or cheese stick.

A water bottle with a straw. One of the signs of milk flow is dry mouth. Holding a water up for your partner to sip with no hands is a big help in the hydration game.

If you won't be able to be around for the day, try to leave these pillows/snacks/fresh water in your partner's common nursing zones or preprepped in the fridge.

If you spot your partner doing a full-body breastfeeding claw—leaning over the baby with their shoulders up to their ears—it is best to adjust them by asking if you can place a pillow here or a blanket there to bring your pair into alignment. You can also try to help unhunch their shoulders with a shoulder rub or heating pad. You should refrain from verbal corrections: your partner is working very hard and it is stressful and they will take it out on you.

Once you have a good latch, I recommend putting your feet up and leaning back. Notice: How does my body feel? Did my baby's latch change?

If so, use micromovements to get back to a good latch.

Now remove your chest-supporting/taco hand. Did that change your latch?

You are now using gravity to hold your baby close. This not only helps you stay more comfortable but lets your baby relax into the feeding and not grab with their mouth for fear of falling away from the breast. You also now have free hands to take a drink of water, online shop, or reposition your baby's lips or jaw, if needed.

If your baby often pops off the breast or you have a very fast letdown lean back even further. You can absolutely nurse a baby all the way flat on your back if your flow is very high.

Side lying

Side lying is a little bit tricky with newborns because it is a hard angle to work with, but it is also lifesaving if your recovery or disability makes lying down more comfortable than sitting. It can also be a game changer for sleep deprivation and dozing while feeding. Lie on your side with your head supported by pillows and a pillow behind your back in the middle of your bed. Remove any extra pillows and fluffy comforters; if you are cold, pull a small blanket over yourself. You will be nursing on your breast that is closest to the mattress. Have a support person place your baby along your body, aligned nose to nipple. You or your support person can hamburger your chest and help baby get a deep latch. If you don't have a support person

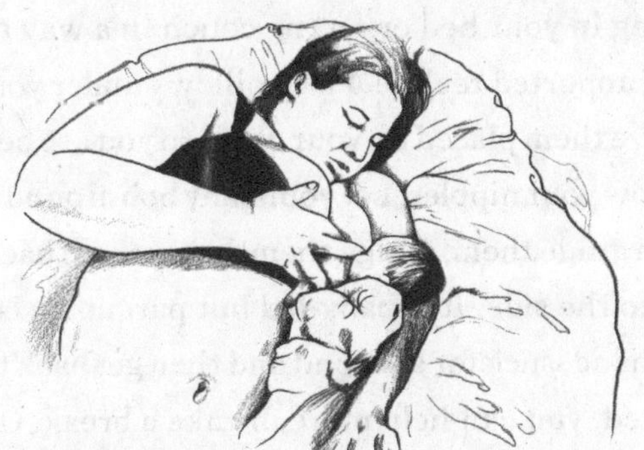

around, you can lay baby onto the bed before you get settled and then scooch them up to you. Forget the chest-supporting hand and use your top arm to help your baby get a deep latch by supporting the base of their head and aiming for a big smoosh.

Once you have a good latch, roll up a blanket or towel to place along your baby's back below the shoulders to help them stay close.

If you are sleepy, make sure you are in the center of the bed, your baby is between you and the edge (not you and a partner or you and a dog), and there are no fluffy blankets or pillows around. Researcher James McKenna has videoed, randomized, and observed a lot of nursing co-sleeping.[11] Turns out, the sleep of a nursing parent is fundamentally different and light when their baby is around. Similarly, babies orient to the smell of milk and move very little while bed sharing. All of this points to dozing while side lying being pretty safe if your family doesn't have other risk factors like drug use or prematurity.

This all becomes much easier after babies are a little bigger and stronger, and most people find this position gets much easier after six weeks. That doesn't mean you shouldn't try it sooner, just that you should know that even if it's tricky in the beginning, it's still a great tool.

BABY-LED POSITIONS

These positions use a baby's natural reflexes so they can latch themselves. While the picture-perfect "breast crawl" right after birth is phenomenally rare, these reflexes are instinctive for most newborns and can be harnessed to help get a surprisingly good latch.

Begin by lying in your bed or on the couch in a way that you would watch TV, in a supported recline. Place pillows under your arms. Scoop your baby or have them placed on your chest so you are belly to belly and your baby is below your nipples. Let your baby bob around and work their way up. You can guide them, nudge them, bring them back to your chest if they flop off to the side. It is baby-led but parent-assisted. They will often land on a hand, suck for a second and then get back to work. If they get too frustrated, you can help more or take a break. Once your baby

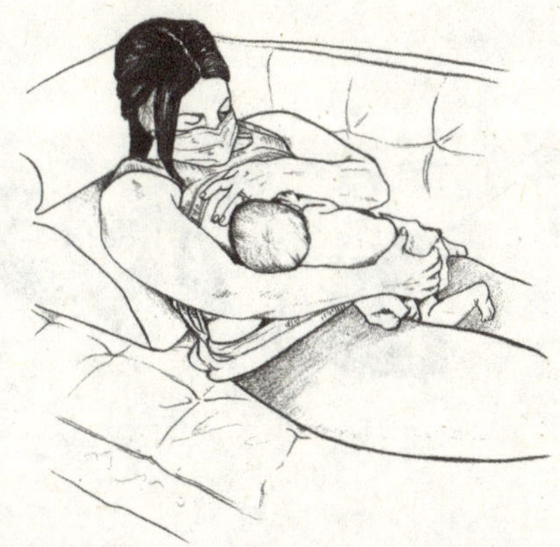

latches, you can adjust your position to make sure it is a good, comfortable latch. Then wrap your arm around so your baby rests in the crook of your arm and settle in.

If you have had a cesarean birth and have a sensitive abdomen, you can adjust this position by reclining more and putting your baby across your chest to work across instead of up. It might also just be something you leave for a few weeks until you have fully healed.

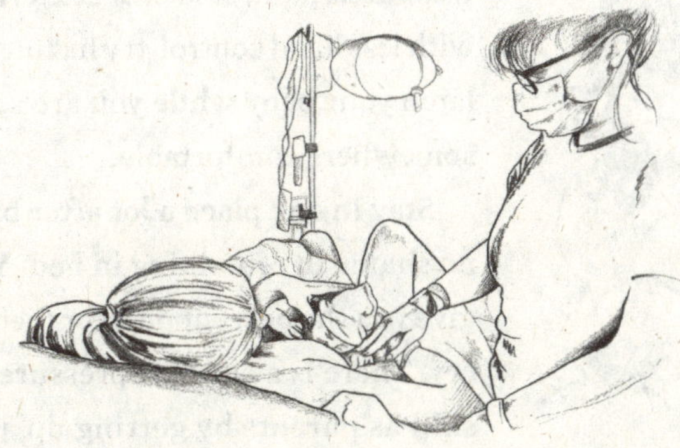

DISABILITY AND POSITIONING

If you are disabled or are having an experience of temporary disability from birthing, you may need specific help figuring out positions that will work for you both.

Try different surfaces and seating. If you have a power chair or a chair that can tilt, you may find that to be an ideal nursing surface because it is

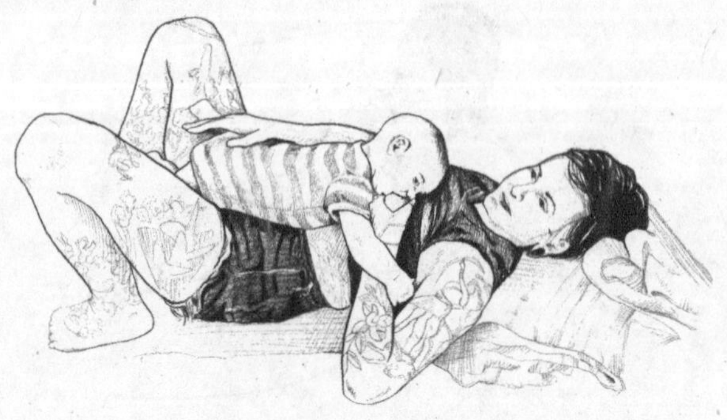

so supportive. Some co-sleeping bassinets can adjust their height easily to position a baby at a comfortable height to slide a baby onto your lap or nursing pillow.

You can use a tool called Kinesio Tape to help shape or support your body. It's a skin-safe tape available at most big box stores or online, which can hold your chest in a comfortable position.

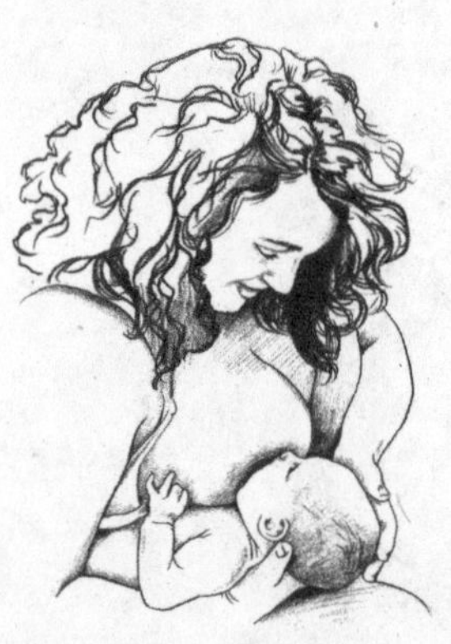

Pillows and towels can assist adaptations for weakness, pain, or lack of dexterity. For people with less hand control, try having someone else latch your baby while you are seated or lying somewhere comfortable.

Stay in one place a lot after birth. There is no shame in remaining in bed. Your bed may give you the best support for feeding or recovery. There is a cultural pressure to prove our skill as parents by getting up and out early, this is a false, and honestly harmful metric of early parenting success. Instead, adopt a plan of "lying in" and staying in the spaces that feel comfortable. If you feel cooped up in your bed but it is most supportive to you, you may want to bring a bed into the living room. Find what works for you and do it, rather than trying to move your body into an imagined ideal of active parenthood.

ASK FOR HELP!

All parents need support and help with feeding in the beginning. Use help to get well set up and to brainstorm adaptations. Try to view feeding as a team sport, and bring in other providers you may have—occupational therapists, physical therapists, etc.—for ideas on how others can support you.

ONE FINAL NOTE

Partners, help with breaks and the reset! If things are getting very chaotic and screamy, no one will do their best work. Suggest taking the baby for a minute and letting your partner reset. They can drink some water, take a few deep breaths and rearrange pillows while you snuggle baby and offer a pacifier or finger to suck on while they calm down, too. These moments are very hard on everyone's nerves, but you can be a regulating force in all the stress.

TROUBLESHOOTING

It is pretty common to run into trouble in these first few weeks. Nursing pain, tongue-ties, high or low production can all interrupt nursing. This system that many assume is fairly straightforward is often a dance of near-constant problem-solving.

ENGORGEMENT AND OTHER EARLY BREASTFEEDING ISSUES

Engorgement is probably the most common breastfeeding complication. Some uncomfortable fullness is just normal to your body's transition of making more milk in the days after birth. While some people definitely have it worse than others, just about everyone experiences some amount of engorgement.

Engorgement is the traffic jam of water to make milk, lymphatic fluid, and swelling of your milk-making tissue that creates a very uncomfortable fullness in your chest. This usually lasts only a few days, beginning around days three to seven as your body goes from making very small amounts of

DANI'S STORY

"I'm still so mad." Dani felt a deep personal drive to breastfeed. Dani had wanted the bond of nursing to give her a closeness with her twin daughters. This thing that only she could do was particularly elusive for Dani as a quadriplegic mom with a spinal cord injury.

The other thing that was elusive for her was help. She had plenty of help with the babies from her husband, who made bottles, changed diapers, and was at her side when they would visit the babies in the NICU. But aside from her husband, Dani had access to almost no support, as her babies were born in April of 2020, in the early days of the COVID-19 pandemic. Dani's family didn't even get a meal train, let alone the level of lactation help she would need to nurse twins. We will never know, but I suspect that if she had been able to have guidance on how to nurse in her wheelchair or bed, she would have been able to meet more of her goals. She didn't even receive much information about pumping. "They handed me this pump, and no one explained anything." Dani triple fed (nursed, pumped, bottle fed; see page 120 for what I recommend doing instead) her NICU nurslings once they got home until unsustainability caught up to her and a wise lactation consultant suggested that since the bonding was what she was after, she could pump and nurse the babies for comfort. Many people experience a deep internal drive to breastfeed and still struggle without nearly as many barriers as Dani had.

Dani cannot simply spring out of bed and run to her children when they need her, and she says, "I really have a grief that I can't do all of the things, and that's not internalized ableism."

Disability is complicated. You can be proudly disabled, know you are an excellent parent, and still feel grief about what you can't do.I have learned so much about parenting from disabled parents like Dani. There is a beautiful truth of parenting that she could grieve over not nursing and be a great mom while not breastfeeding. Because Dani could not have lactation support in her home, she was left to figure things out. And she did figure things out: her daughters are thriving in their matching outfits with their exuberant personalities.

Dani's story is an important reminder to find the positioning that works for your body. Whether you are a disabled parent or a parent who is temporarily disabled from a surgical birth or difficult birth recovery: nurse where you are comfortable and find the ways that make it comfortable for you.

If there is a tool or a position you have found that works for you, I encourage you to use it, even if it doesn't look like anything suggested in this book or elsewhere.

thick milk to making larger amounts of thinner milk. You may have heard this called "milk coming in." I don't use this phrase because I find it confusing. I think it makes people feel like they didn't have milk to begin with. You do, just less, and it's thicker.

To resolve engorgement and get more comfortable, you need to get swelling down and get the excess lymphatic fluid back to where your body can recirculate it.

Step 1: Decrease inflammation

Ice between feedings for twenty minutes with true ice (not a bag of peas) wrapped in a thin towel. With your provider's permission, take ibuprofen.

Step 2: Massage lymphatic fluid out

Use the following lymphatic drainage techniques to engage your lymphatic system and carry excess fluid out of the way.

1. Place a finger above your collarbone two inches from your clavicle, about where a necklace would lie in the triangle of your neck and collarbone. Gently rub ten little circles. It will feel like you aren't doing anything. That's fine; I promise that you are. Now find the place where your armpit meets your breast. Think about the area that peeks out of the straps of a swimsuit, the "chub" as I call it. Rub ten small circles here to engage your lymph nodes.

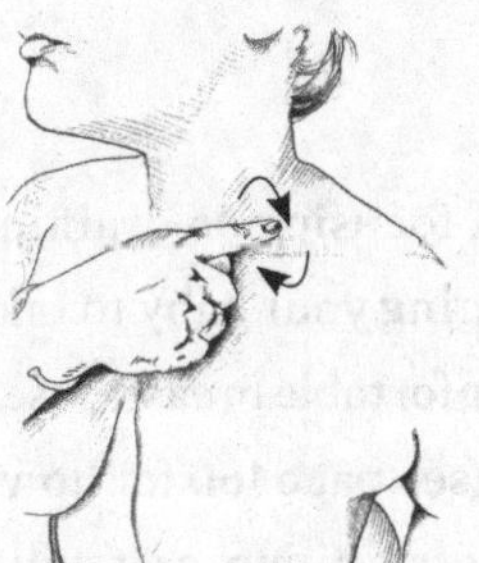

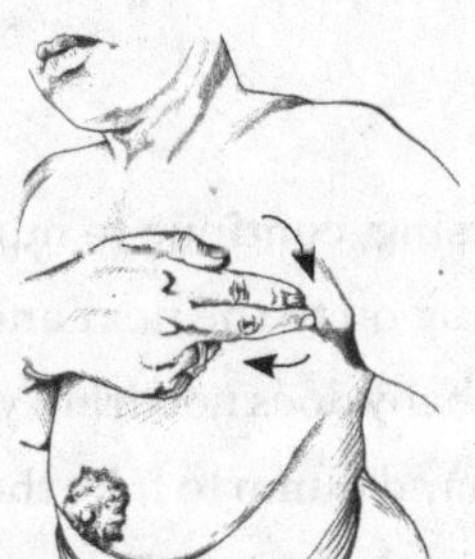

2. Lie back and lift your breast up off the chest wall. Think of this like lifting a sprained ankle to drain fluid. With both hands lift the breast off the chest wall and count to thirty. You may want to ask for someone's help with this if you have large breasts or find the position awkward.

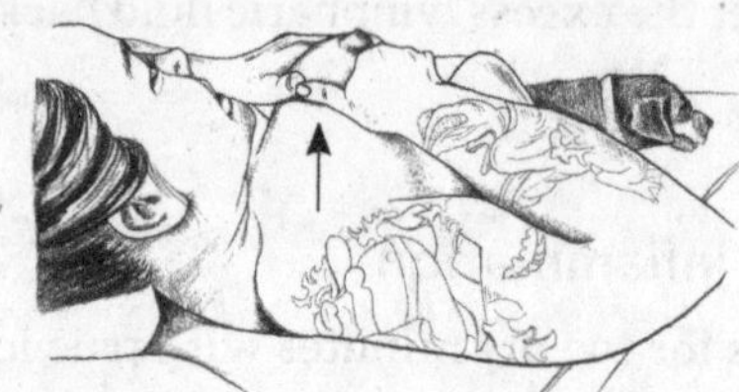

3. Gently massage toward the armpit. Remember, this is glandular tissue, not muscle: be respectful. With your palms or the side of your hand sweep up toward your armpits. Think of this like scraping brownie batter from a bowl, working your way around the breast to sweep it all. Oil can help you glide over the skin comfortably, but don't use more pressure than you would use petting a cat.

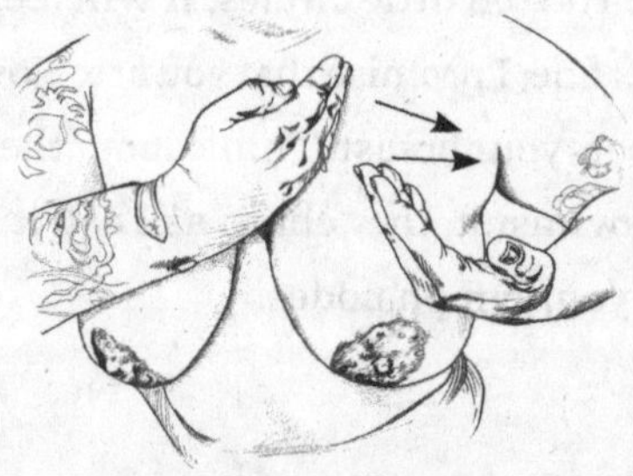

If you are nursing, continue to nurse on cue, focusing on draining one side before moving on to the next and encouraging your baby to take full feedings. If your baby does not drain your uncomfortable breasts, use hand expression or a hand pump to take the edge off (see page 160 for how to do it), but not to drain the breast. Do not use an electric pump, as it will stimulate more swelling and milk production.

If you are exclusively pumping, use your electric pump as you have been and drain your breasts, but do not continue pumping beyond that. Use massage to stay comfortable between scheduled pumping sessions.

NIPPLE EVERSION, LATCH, AND ENGORGEMENT

We talked about nipples a bit on page 93. Nipples are as varied as people themselves. Some nipples are just harder to latch onto than others; some people just have naturally flat or inverted nipples. People with connective tissue disabilities like Ehlers-Danlos syndrome may have soft, stretchy nipple tissue. Engorgement can make all of these things more challenging by making the tissue around your nipple swollen. To help with this, you can use massage to push that fluid back and create a nipple that's easier to latch onto. You may also need to use a nipple shield (see page 106 for how these work and how to put them on).

Reverse pressure softening

Often fluids from birth or engorgement can make latching your baby really hard. This method is a tool to make your nipple stick out more to get a better latch. It moves fluid away from the nipple so it stands up until your baby is comfortably latched.

The Claw: With your fingers facing you, make a claw by bending your fingertips toward each other. Push that claw firmly into your breast around your nipple, hold it there, and count to thirty.

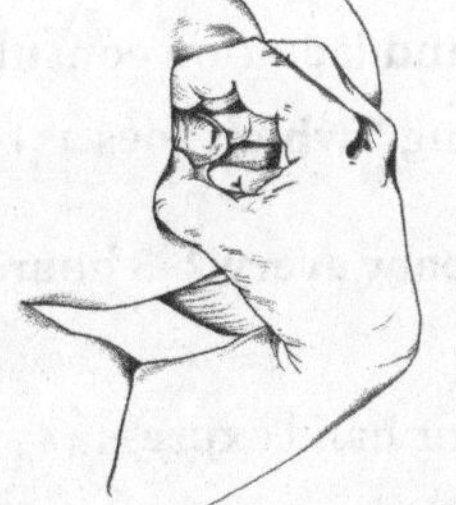

The Flight Attendant: If you have long nails and the Claw isn't a good fit, try "the Flight Attendant" instead. Hold two fingers up on each hand like you are directing passengers to the exit rows on an airplane. Press your fingers flat against your breast on either side of your nipple, parallel to one another, pointing to your toes. Then go the other direction so each set of fingers is pointing at the opposite armpit. Hold each direction firmly for thirty seconds.

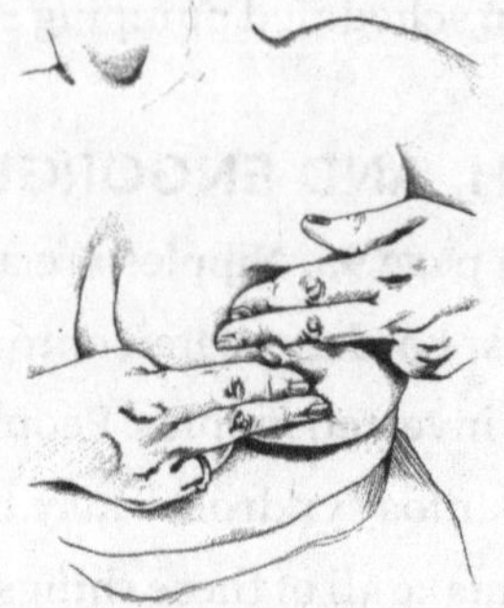

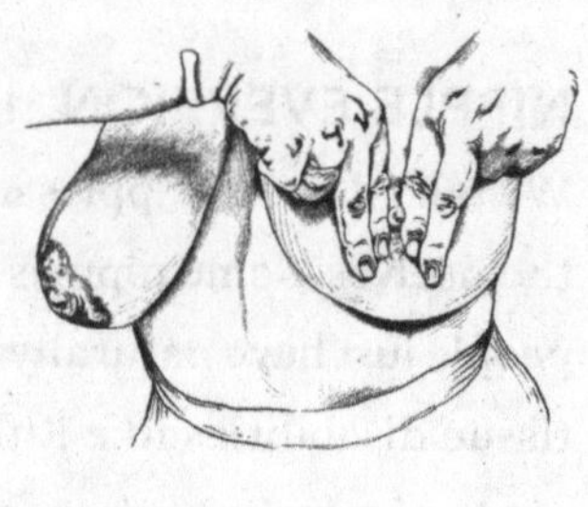

OTHER COMMON BUMPS IN YOUR NURSING ROAD

Slow or no weight gain

When a baby isn't gaining weight, we need to supplement their diet with pumped milk, donor milk, or formula to keep them healthy while we figure out what the root cause is. If we give a baby an outside food source, then the nursing person misses out on those hormone spikes that set the right amount of milk production for your baby. This means that in order to maintain milk production while we solve the problem, a nursing parent ideally expresses milk eight to twelve times per day in the first six weeks.

Doctors and lactation consultants may recommend something called "triple feeding," which goes as below:

- Wake baby every 2–3 hours
- Nurse
- Pump or hand express
- Offer bottle
- Repeat at 2- to 3-hour mark based on the START of the last feeding.

This system is very effective at resolving the slow weight gain but leaves a parent with effectively no sleep with the added stress of worrying. I have worked with countless families to unravel the web they are left in from triple feeding. It just isn't sustainable beyond a day or two. If your baby has a tongue-tie (page 46), or a more complex feeding issue that your lactation team doesn't think will be resolved within a few days, I recommend this instead:

- Offer nursing at two good times per 24 hours. Aim for a time when you and your baby are calm, relatively well rested, and not overly hungry.
- Pump and paced bottle feed all other feedings (6–10 per day).
- If your baby is not nursing effectively at all, you will need to pump and bottle feed after your two nursing sessions, which while frustrating, is more manageable than twelve.

Once your baby's feeding-based medical issue is resolved, you should be cleared to return to a more sustainable and natural feeding rhythm and add more nursings. If your baby had an effective feeding that drained your breasts and your baby is giving fullness cues, there is no need to pump after that feeding. (See page 193 on decoding a feeding.)

Pain in nursing

Another reason why we need to step in on nursing and offer bottles is pain. If you are in pain with nursing, or nursing is causing damage, you need to do something until you get help. This help might be a tongue-tie revision (page 48), bodywork for your baby (page 57), or seeing a lactation professional to work on latch.

HOW TO SURVIVE PAINFUL NURSING UNTIL YOU CAN GET HELP

Sometimes when you have significant nursing pain it takes time to resolve the issue. It's important to make a sustainable plan while you see a lactation professional/revise a tongue-tie/work through body asymmetries.

If you feel overwhelmed, try to break time up into smaller chunks. What is our plan for the night? What feels doable today? Or even, what feels manageable at this feeding. One feeding at a time. One day at a time. One week at a time.

EARLY PUMPING TO ASSIST WITH PAIN OR SUPPLEMENTATION

Early pumping can add another complicating variable. It can also be a very helpful tool to prevent tissue damage whilst you wait to get help. You can skip a feeding, pump and offer a paced bottle to give your nipples a break.

IF YOUR BABY NEEDS SUPPLEMENTATION

UNTIL MILK TRANSITION

From days one through five or until your milk transition occurs, hand expression is often more effective than pumping because of the small volumes and stickiness of colostrum (early milk). This milk can be expressed right into a spoon and tipped into a baby's mouth. If your medical team feels that your baby needs more milk (formula or donor milk) on top of this, it can be given via a syringe or bottle. You can also use a pump during this time just for stimulation if you prefer that to hand expressing, but it can be hard to give that milk to baby. This is FINE. It is okay to treat pumping like going to the gym and working out your body to bring on a milk transition and to rely on other calorie sources to feed your baby.

AFTER MILK TRANSITION

Once milk has transitioned and is thinner, it can be more easily expressed by a pump. Using hand expression can help make pumping more effective (page 160), and using lymphatic drainage techniques (page 117) can help reduce the risk of engorgement. Remember that the goal is to use the pump to protect production while letting the tissue of your nipples rest and heal. It's important that the pump only be turned up to a suction level that is comfortable but effective—like "Yup, I feel that. It's comfortable, any higher would be uncomfortable"—your flanges fit well (page 155), and that you lubricate your flanges. If pumping hurts no matter the flange size and suction, you may want to just hand express.

NIPPLE CARE

While your nipples are healing, remember: milk and moisture. After any nursing or expressing, rub in a few drops of your own milk followed by a goop barrier (Aquaphor, coconut oil, nipple cream, etc.) and if bumping into things/hugs/kicks/your clothes hurt your nipple, use a hydrogel, Silverette, or if you are feeling hippy-dippy, clean seashell to create a barrier between your nipples and the world.

MOOD AND PAIN

Pain and difficulty nursing are risk factors for and often cause postpartum mood disorders. It doesn't help that this early painful nursing also tends to fall right in the middle of your hormone transition, which is already a highly emotional time. It's common to feel like a failure (you're not; these things happen and are out of your control) or like nothing will ever change (they will; babies are very malleable and every day is a little different from the last). Try to make sure you are getting some sleep (protected sleep, see page 254), and if you can't sleep or don't feel better after sleeping, it's a good idea to check in with your primary care provider or call the twenty-four-hour birth line from your birthing provider and ask for help. Feeding babies is very complex, and it can feel like a litmus test for who we are as parents. Don't let that get you; you are a great parent while you navigate what life throws your way and find the best way for your family to feed this baby.

To my tough ones out there: Nursing through pain doesn't help anyone. If your latch looks good and you are in pain, there is an underlying cause and finding this cause is what will resolve the pain. Tissue and nerve damage from pushing through pain tends to make things worse. Also, you are a person, and I like you, and you shouldn't push through painful things (except birth, there's not much we can do about that one).

Goals while healing from painful nursing:

- Rest, recovery, breaks from pain
- 8–12 expressions per 24 hours to protect production (this can be nursing, pumping, or hand expression)
- Baby eating enough per pediatrician's recommended volumes (this can be formula, donor milk, or pumped milk)
- Nursing 2+ times per 24 hours to preserve nursing reflexes and work on skills
- Paced bottle feeding for slow flow and skill building

Protocol for surviving feeding difficulties

STEP 1: SLEEP

Ask a support person or partner to offer a bottle and go to bed for four to six hours of protected sleep. Do a good expressing session, eat a snack, put on cozy pajamas, white noise, earplugs, an eye mask and get into bed. This sleep will not have a meaningful impact on milk production long-term and will help you have the clarity and stamina to make good decisions going forward.

STEP 2: TRY CUE-BASED FEEDING

Take twelve to twenty-four hours to let your baby wake themselves for feedings. If they do not wake for eight to twelve feedings in twenty-four hours, you know that you need to return to clock-based feedings. If they do reliably wake and eat well eight to twelve times per day, we know that their weight and nervous system can be trusted to continue moving forward. If you are in pain but want to continue with nursing, offer two nursings per day and do cue-based bottle feedings until the cause of your nursing troubles has been resolved.

STEP 3: WATCH FOR FULLNESS CUES

Feed your baby not based on volume but based on fullness. (See page 194 on baby fullness cues.) Watch these cues during bottle feeding and nursing. At what point in a bottle does your baby reach full, milk-drunk status? How does your chest feel when your baby reaches that same point? Just observe for now. If your baby just can't seem to get full enough from nursing, talk to a lactation consultant to figure out why. It could be a tongue-tie, insufficient suck, low production, etc. This period of observation will help your team understand what is going on and made a plan.

If you are in pain when nursing, skip this and remain at the two nursings, six-pumping phase until pain cause has been identified and resolved.

STEP 4: FADE DOWN THE PUMPING

As you have more bandwidth for nursing and your baby is more reliably waking for nursing and getting a full intake, you can fade out the pumping and bottles until just one cycle of pumping and bottles remains. I recommend leaving this one for other caregiver bonding or to keep the flexibility of bottle feeding later on when you want to go see a movie.

The trick to figuring out supplementation without impacting production is to understand where your point of diminishing return is (see page 236 for how to work this out). Staying ahead of where that line is will keep production up, whereas crossing it regularly will bring production down. In most cases, expressing will bring production back up when needed.

LUMPS, BUMPS, AND PLUGS

While engorgement and latching difficulties are very common in the first week of nursing, other challenges crop up at different times for different people. It is normal to need help at various points in nursing, and acting quickly when you notice a persistent lump or sore or hot red area is important.

Breast tissue is lumpy by nature. Understanding your baseline is super important, both for lactation and for lifelong cancer monitoring. You may find that while lactating you get more persistent lumps and what are commonly thought of as "plugged ducts."

The lump you feel in the breast is not actually a clog; ducts are microscopic at that point in the breast. What you are feeling is a buildup, or as brilliant IBCLC and breast surgeon Katrina Mitchell, MD, IBCLC, explains it, a traffic jam.[12] This can be swelling in the tissue around the duct, or a knot of fascia around the duct.

Monitoring

If you notice a bump, and if it also has a change in skin color or texture, touch base with your doctor. If a lump lasts more than a week, you should ask for an ultrasound in case cancer screening is indicated.

Reduce swelling

Dr. Mitchell helped me understand swelling and plugged ducts in a whole new way. As I mentioned before, she compares them to a traffic jam. In order to move the milk traffic through, you cannot just force it; you have to change the traffic pattern. This is done in a few ways: widening the ducts by reducing the swelling around them so they can open up, reducing the bacteria that may be blocking milk flow, reducing milk flow to balance the system, or by making the milk easier to move emulsifying it.

WIDEN THE ROAD (DUCT):

Lymphatic drainage. If you have a plug that is due to a buildup of fluid around the ducts (especially likely if you are newly postpartum), try this simple lymphatic drainage technique several times throughout the day. Remember that this tissue is made of glands, not muscle. So treat it gently.

- 10 small circles with your finger in the soft triangle over the collarbone, where a necklace would hit.
- 10 small circles with your finger in the lymphatic hub in your armpit in the "chub" (a.k.a. the space between your bra strap and armpit).
- With the back of your hand and oil or lotion, sweep around your chest towards the arm pit like you are scraping brownie batter from a bowl. This should be like petting a cat, not deep tissue massage.

Elevation. Lying on your back, lift your breast up off the chest wall and hold it there for a minute. This can help clear a way to open up that bridge. You may also find that using rolled-up towels or receiving blankets can help you elevate large breasts to comfortably sleep without smooshing the affected area.

If you have a persistently uncomfortable plug or swollen area, you may want to access ultrasound. Unlike vibration from an electric toothbrush or vibrator, ultrasound has been shown to more gently treat these areas without causing damage. This can be done by a doctor or physical therapist.

The details of these techniques are on page 131.

Expression. Be careful with expression. If you are nursing, use your baby to express milk instead of the pump. If your baby isn't nursing well or you

are exclusively pumping, use the pump on a comfortable setting, and only until the breast softens. Too much suction from a pump can draw swelling back into the breast and continue the cycle. These areas of inflammation are caused by overproducing milk and not allowing your body to find a comfortable supply and demand. Continuing to increase demand to "keep your breasts empty" can actually make this much worse.

Do not go full blast to pull the clog out while jamming away at the clog with a deep tissue massage. These common interventions often make things worse and can cause a dreadful but amusingly named *flegmon*, or bunch of inflamed and damaged tissue. It can feel like you aren't doing much, but these gentle techniques are more effective and less likely to cause damage. I know its hard, but when it comes to plugged ducts and mastitis, I'm going to ask you to do less. Get into bed and rest. Nurse or pump as you usually do.

Ice and NSAIDs. Once you have done lymphatic drainage and expression, you may want to ice the duct to reduce any swelling in the actual tissue that can be caused by all this activity. You'll want true ice; no frozen peas. Some great ice packs include a newborn diaper full of water and then frozen, a dedicated ice pack for athletes or injury, or a bag of ice wrapped in a towel to protect your skin. Ten minutes of ice every hour should be fine, then leave your tissues alone for a while and only begin the process again if the lump reappears or persists.

If your breast is so swollen that milk won't come out, do even less. Do lymphatic drainage and use NSAIDs to stay comfortable, but mostly rest. Try not to panic and just go to bed. Do not keep trying to feed and pump on that side. Call your doctor, go to bed, and let your immune system work.

Galactocele

A galactocele is a cyst-like collection of milk behind a duct that has been narrowed by swelling or bacterial overgrowth. This may feel like a large painful lump and can develop into mastitis. Remember that you cannot massage the milk through the narrowed path in front of it. You have to widen the path by reducing swelling. If you suspect a galactocele, get in touch with your birth provider and have them monitor you to see if antibiotics are needed or if the galactocele needs to be drained surgically.

Blebs

Sometimes a clog goes all the way to the nipple. You may notice an (often painful) white spot on the outlets of your nipple or skin covering one outlet like a blister. This is sometimes caused by milk coagulating (congealing) all the way to the tip of a nipple or swelling or bacteria blocking the duct. You should use the same lymphatic drainage techniques and ask your doctor about a topical steroid (which is safe for nursing). It may also help to take a lecithin supplement to emulsify milk so it can clear more easily through the narrowed duct. It is no longer recommended to "unroof" or soak a bleb which can cause more swelling and introduce bacteria.

Mastitis

Mastitis is . . . the worst. It's extremely common, affecting about one in four breastfeeding people in the first twenty-six weeks after a pregnancy. Mastitis is an infection in the breast that is diagnosed and categorized by its symptoms:

- Breast pain
- Redness
- A persistent lump
- Swelling
- Hot to the touch
- Fever
- Chills
- Aches
- "Flu-like symptoms"

It can range from a warm lump in the breast to feeling like having the flu after being hit by a truck while your breasts slowly turn to hot stone.

There are new theories about what causes mastitis as we come to learn more about the importance of the microbiome. It seems that mastitis can be genetic or be caused by less direct nursing (a.k.a. pumping or using a shield) because it changes the bacterial exchange between a nursing person and a baby. It is worsened by stress and commonly caused by overproduction or disruptions in a nursing feedback loop.

While mastitis can generalize to a whole breast or both breasts, there is usually one offending duct with a firm blockage.

Inflammatory mastitis is caused by swelling in the tissue that causes blockage to the ducts. While very uncomfortable, this kind of mastitis will resolve with lymphatic drainage and *lots of rest*. You should check in with your provider to determine if your mastitis is inflammatory and have them monitor you closely in case it progresses to bacterial mastitis.

Bacterial mastitis should be flagged if you develop a fever or tachycardia (racing pulse). This is a bacterial infection caused by an overgrowth of bacteria in the ducts. This is not caused by bacteria in your environment so there is no need to sanitize everything; good hand washing will do. Unlike inflammatory mastitis, you should not try to treat bacterial mastitis on your own and should contact your provider for treatment.

Mastitis treatment

While most people are able to treat their mastitis on their own, the first thing you want to do is check in with your provider. If you have a fever, dust off that twenty-four-hour call line from late pregnancy and use it. Your provider will know if it's safe to take ibuprofen and may call in some antibiotics to take if the infection doesn't start to resolve. They also need to be aware of what's going on in case they need to rule out an abscess (a very serious infection that needs to be surgically drained to prevent spreading).

To treat inflammatory mastitis yourself, and using the road analogy from before, we need to move traffic jammed by swelling in the tissue. The way to get things moving is to make the road wider by doing lymphatic drainage (both to move fluid and help your body carry away bacteria) and getting the swelling down by using ice and ibuprofen. Ask your team what symptoms to watch for to know if things are improving or if it is time for clinical intervention and in person monitoring.

Just like with a sprained ankle, you are going to use the RICE method for mastitis.

REST. is extremely important. Mastitis can get very serious and result in hospitalization. This is no time for your partner to go to a pickup game of basketball. Call in your support network and get into bed. The only thing that is a priority for the next 48 hours is resting and decreasing swelling. If other people can pitch in with childcare and bring your baby to you for feedings all the better. Get into bed and stay there.

ICE. True ice is a great way to reduce inflammation. Wrap a bag of ice in a kitchen towel and place it on the affected area. Don't exceed twenty minutes.

IBUPROFEN. If considered safe for you by your care provider, this can help keep your fever down and help reduce inflammation.

COMPRESSION. If you are pumping, use gentle compression to mimic nursing and help your body move milk effectively. Do not aggressively massage squeeze your breasts. Use hand expression or gentle hands on pumping and do not pump excessively.

If your symptoms do not resolve within forty-eight hours (twenty-four on antibiotics), it is time to see a provider in person. Mastitis can evolve into an abscess or rarely, sepsis (a bacterial infection that gets into other body systems), which can be very dangerous.

ELEVATION. While this one sounds strange, use the lift-up technique on page 126 by either lifting your breast or having someone else lift your breast while you lie flat and hold it up for a few minutes. Pair this with the other lymphatic drainage techniques to reduce swelling. Remember, be gentle. Like petting a cat.

OTHER THINGS THAT MAY HELP

Stay hydrated. Your immune system needs hydration to work. Make sure to keep your water bottle full and your urine light.

Ultrasound. This uses ultrasound waves to break up fat and move lymphatic fluid to get your system flowing again and resolve infection. Ask your providers if there is anyone in your area who does this.

Kinesio Tape. If your breast is painful in some positions and comfortable in others, you can use Kinesio Tape (a skin-safe tape available at most big box stores or online) to hold your chest in a comfortable position that will also allow your lymph and fluid to drain more effectively.

PREVENTION FOR RECURRENT MASTITIS/LUMPS

For some reason, some people are just more prone to mastitis than others. If you are someone who has recurrent mastitis, try to recognize the early signs as well as use preventative measures.

Thoughtful drainage. You will need to be more careful about how often and how well you drain your breasts. Work with a lactation consultant to bring production down to see if that helps.

Lecithin and probiotics. Try a probiotic that contains *L. fermentum* or, preferably, *L. salivarius* for prevention, add a lethecin supplement. This dietary supplement is an emulsifier found in favorite foods all over the grocery store. An emulsifier is something that helps fats bind to water (like salad dressing). If you have very frequent clogs (more than once a month) you may just have sticky, fatty milk. This supplement can help your milk be less sticky and flow more easily. Generally, it is derived from soy or sunflowers.

Resolve the underlying cause. The recurrent mastitis could be caused by an antibiotic-resistant bacteria. Ask for a milk culture to rule out bacteria like MRSA-resistant CoNS.

Work with a lactation professional to make sure your pump works well, your baby doesn't have any oral ties and that your latch looks good to resolve the underlying cause of the mastitis.

HOW TO MANAGE A LEAKY CHEST

Postpartum is a regrettably damp and leaky time. Between the night sweats, bleeding, and milk leakage from you or baby . . . I recommend buying an extra set of sheets. You can layer mattress cover–sheet–mattress cover–sheet or towel–sheet–towel–sheet on your and baby's bed to make middle-of-the-night sheet changes more doable.

As far as the leaky-chest situation goes, here are a few things that may help.

Push back

Direct pressure into the nipple and breast can help tell your body "Hey, stop it. We aren't flowing right now." This is done by pushing directly back into the chest wall with the flat palm of your hand and counting to thirty. If you happen to be in a meeting or grocery store, you can achieve the same effect by crossing your arms over your chest and pushing back.

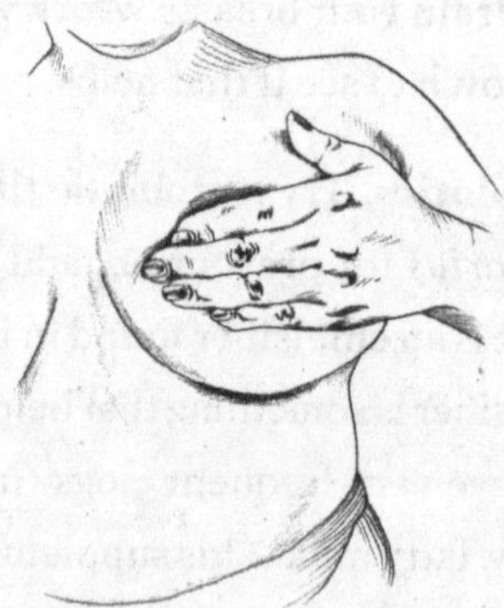

Stack nursing pads

Sleep bras that offer little in the support department but hold nursing pads in place are a big help with bed-wetting issues. You can layer cotton nursing pads followed by a disposable nursing pad at the back to double or triple absorbency while you are sleeping.

Passive-collection inserts

If you predominantly leak on one side while nursing on the other, you can use a collection attachment or passive pump while you nurse. Some of these are firm plastic cups that you tuck into your bra, while another is a silicone suction bulb that you attach with negative pressure. Holding this in place with a pumping bra can help you reduce spills. You can also wear a collection insert throughout the day if you are an all-day leaker. It is important to empty these cups every hour or two. You can store that milk and wash the cups with hot soapy water. These cups are held close to your body and are thus kept very warm. This is a bacterial happy place, so more washing caution is needed than with room-temperature milk storage.

Acceptance

At some point you just accept this a leaky time. This is the Renaissance-painting phase of life, and there is only so much you can do about it. Buy extra shirts that fit nicely to keep in your bag and glamorously tuck cloth diapers into your shirt while you hang around the house.

HOW TO MANAGE OVERSUPPLY[13]

We live in a culture of more is MORE! If you are experiencing oversupply, you know the truth: more milk can cause more problems. The goal in milk production is a harmonious balance where you have enough milk to feed your baby/babies. Not too much, not too little.

Some people are just prone to overproduction because of their genetics; others experience oversupply from overstimulation in early nursing or pumping. Pumping excessively (*excess* here really differs person to person, but after all or most feedings would apply) can also put someone in a state of overproduction.

Signs and symptoms of overproduction

UNCOMFORTABLY FULL AND LEAKING BETWEEN FEEDINGS

If your production and your baby are out of sync then your body may hurt between feedings as though your body is screaming: *BUT I HAVE MORE BABIES TO FEED!* It doesn't, and your body needs to chill.

FREQUENT PLUGGED DUCTS OR MASTITIS

If your chest is constantly full, this can lead to the conditions that cause mastitis. Your baby may also get full before they drain your breast well, leaving a backup of milk that can feel like a plug. Refer back to page 129 for mastitis treatment.

NIPPLE BLEBS

These little plugs at the very tip of the nipple are coagulated milk that can create a plug in a duct. They are very uncomfortable and can be treated with lethecin and a steroid cream. Refer back to page 128 for bleb treatment.

VASOSPASM

So much milk trying to move through your chest can cause a circulation issue called *vasospasm*. This is also caused by nerve damage from a poor latch. Vasospasm can cause changes in color to the nipple, which may turn white or purple/blue. It can also cause shooting pains back into the breast tissue. For help with latch issues, see page 103.

FOREMILK/HINDMILK IMBALANCE AND WHAT IT MEANS FOR FEEDING

As milk moves through ducts, the thinner, higher-sugar milk moves first, leaving the higher-fat milk to move towards the end of the feeding. If you are nursing or pumping and produce more milk than your baby can eat, they often get an imbalance of lactose to fat and protein. The best clue is bright green mucus-y poop. While these individual symptoms can be treated, to reduce them overall, you will need to bring down production. This is done very gradually by reducing the demand for milk by pumping or nursing less. If you are pumping between feedings to drain your breasts, you will want to gradually pump less and less, getting to where your breasts will stay full but comfortable. Reducing production requires you to do some close

body listening and find those thresholds of where you are developing plugs or mastitis, and working to balance supply while not getting an infection.

Start by reducing pumping time by five minutes. Use lymphatic massage techniques to reduce fluid and plugs without fully softening your chest. After a week or so, you should get consistently more comfortable and be able to reduce by another five minutes. Then after a few weeks, drop any extra pumping sessions. If a pumping session is replacing a nursing, leave it as is. If it is in addition to nursing, try to reduce it.

Try this flow of massages to get comfortable while leaving your chest not fully drained:

- Push with flat palms directly back into your chest wall. Not so firmly that it hurts, just enough to feel pressure. Hold for thirty seconds.
- Lean back, ideally flat on your back, and lift your breast up off your chest wall. This allows some of that swelling to drain back. Hold up for thirty seconds.
- Using a nice massage oil, like coconut oil, massage in big sweeps back towards your armpit. This should help move some of the swelling back.
- Now, feed your baby or pump.

If you are still uncomfortably full after, try using a silicon passive pump to "take the edge off" without stimulating milk production too much. Apply just enough pressure to keep the pump on, or use a hands-free pumping bra to hold on while you massage.

If pumping is not part of the reason for your oversupply, you may just be predisposed to the condition. For this, you will want to use a tool called *block feeding*. Before you start block feeding, check in with a lactation provider who can confirm your oversupply and monitor your health for mastitis and your baby's weight gain. Give yourself forty-eight hours to see if it's working; if it isn't, you may need to bring in other tools.

Body-based block feeding

Nurse on one side for as many feeds as it takes to feel soft on the side. Leave the other side as full as possible without being in pain or developing clogs/ mastitis. Use massage, hand expression, or a passive pump on your full side to stay comfortable before it is time to feed on that side again.

Clock-based block feeding

If you find it hard to tell when your chest is soft, you will want to use the clock as a guide. During the day, feed your baby on the same side every time you nurse within a three-hour block before switching to the other side. As many feeds as they desire, just go back to that same side. Use massage, passive pumping, and hand expression to keep that side comfortable while full. After three hours, switch. At night, however, feed in whatever way works best and is comfortable enough to get back to sleep.

This system works by leaving a breast full, which stretches out your milk-making receptors so that your lactating tissue can't receive the signal to make more milk.

If after forty-eight hours of block feeding there is no change in comfort or milk production, you should talk to your medical team about prescription options. Your doctor may use either pseudoephedrine (we don't know why this over-the-counter allergy medication drops milk production, but it does) or a dopamine agonist like cabergoline.

Full-drainage block feeding

If the other tools are not working, you may want to consider full-drainage block feeding. In some case studies, people have found success with this method over other styles for rebalancing production.[14] This is done by pumping both sides until they are as softened and drained as possible. This can take thirty minutes to an hour. When you see a significant decrease in flow and feel softer or less heavy, then offer nursing to your baby. Nurse on cue using the clock to block feed. This can help your body get a full reset more quickly or easily than a gradual block feeding. You can repeat this process any time you notice an oversupply redeveloping.

MANAGING FEEDING WITH OVERSUPPLY

Lean back

The first line of support in managing oversupply is gravity. By leaning back, your baby will have better control of milk flow. Instead of gulping milk down like a beer funnel, your baby has the option to open their mouth and let excess milk run off. This will also help your baby breathe normally while nursing, which should help with gas and reflux.

Take your regular latch somewhere where you can lie down, like your couch or bed. Once your baby is latched, lean as far back as you comfortably can so your baby is uphill from your milk flow.

Let milk run off

You can also let some of your first, fastest milk run off a bit. You'll need to also use other strategies to reduce production, but if your first priority is helping your baby get more comfortable, this can help. Hand express until you have a letdown and let that milk just run off into a towel or bottle and then latch your baby. This milk is absolutely fine to save and feed to your baby. Do not use a pump to do this, it will make the problem worse.

SHUTTING DOWN MILK PRODUCTION

There are some circumstances where you know you do not plan to provide your milk for your baby. This might be an external reason like the needing to take a medication that's incompatible with lactation, or an internal one like gender dysphoria or just not wanting to. All reasons to not make milk are good reasons to not make milk. It is your body, you get to chose what you want to do with it. Shutting down milk production is known as "drying off."

While it is ideal to slowly and gradually shut down milk production, sometimes your circumstances mean you need to do so in a hurry.

1. Use as little expression as possible to stay comfortable and healthy. Using a hand pump, hand expression, and lymphatic drainage, express enough milk to keep from getting mastitis and to be able to rest comfortably.
2. Talk to your care provider about herbs and drugs. The most commonly used tools are sage, pseudoephedrine (decongestant), or birth control. All of these have side effects and should be used carefully and with guidance from someone who knows what else you are taking.

CHAPTER 6

BOTTLE FEEDING

Most of us bottle feed our babies. You may be exclusively bottle feeding, or you may be primarily nursing but aspire to go to the movies one time in the next year. Bottles are a great tool for sharing the work of baby feeding, teaching sucking skills, and diversifying your baby's comforting strategies.

CHOOSING A BOTTLE

There are bottles that look like a breast, bottles with vacuum bags, and mixed bottle sets for sampling. However, if offered at the right developmental moment (under six weeks of age) most babies will take most bottles.

Start with a small number of small bottles, four ounces or smaller. Early on, your baby won't need an eight-ounce bottle. Some babies never need an eight-ounce bottle. If you are exclusively bottle feeding, you will want four to twelve bottles depending on how often you will wash them/minimalism/budget. If you are breastfeeding, you can start with two and then buy more as needed.

Look for the bottle that fits your hand best so you can hold it like a pencil. I find that a narrow-neck bottle approximates a good latch, which is important for all babies. They are also the easiest to hold and pace.

If you have weakness in your grip strength you should also factor in comfortable angles and sizes for your hands or add products like sleeves or easy hold straps to help you bottle feed.

JULIETTE'S STORY

Juliette is the kind of woman who plans elaborate professional photo shoots for herself. She is studious and curious and has fierce in her maternal energy. She knows what she wants, and she likes to plan. "With Caleb I made what felt like an easy informed decision to breastfeed." Juliette was logical; the lactation consultant and newborn-care class never mentioned formula, breast milk is "better," so she set out to breastfeed. After an unexpected cesarean birth, though, Juliette's milk transitioned slowly. "The mental toll of worrying about my baby losing weight and not producing enough milk was extremely stressful." Caleb was a super sweet baby when he wasn't crying for hours on end for no apparent reason. Juliette studiously tried everything, she imported European formula, bought fancy sleep sacks: anything to make him more comfortable. This colicky time was likely due to the fact that Caleb is autistic. As is common with autistic newborns, he had sensory needs that he couldn't work through or communicate at such a young age. At six to nine months, his personality started to shine through, "He loved to open and close things, flip through pages, and organize flash cards, yes, as an infant."

When Juliette became unexpectedly pregnant with her second, she made a different plan. Finding neurodiversity-affirming childcare for nonspeaking autistic kids is extremely challenging. Juliette developed Bell's palsy in pregnancy and was in constant pain. It was a very difficult time. "I knew I had to do things differently with Chloe, so I decided to not initiate nursing." Knowing that a new baby in the house would be a huge change for her son, Juliette needed another caregiver to be able to feed the new baby and knew that she did not want to pump. This time, she selected a reliable American brand to avoid supply-chain issues. After a successful VBAC (vaginal birth after cesarean) she very much wanted, she told the lactation consultant that she would be exclusively formula feeding. "I didn't express at all. It was really painful, but I let things be, and after two weeks, I dried up." People asked if she was worried about having the same bond with Chloe. "I felt like we actually had more interactive time together. To me, there was no downside to not chest-feeding Chloe. I wasn't concerned about her weight and growth. There was zero anxiety around making sure she was fed and healthy."

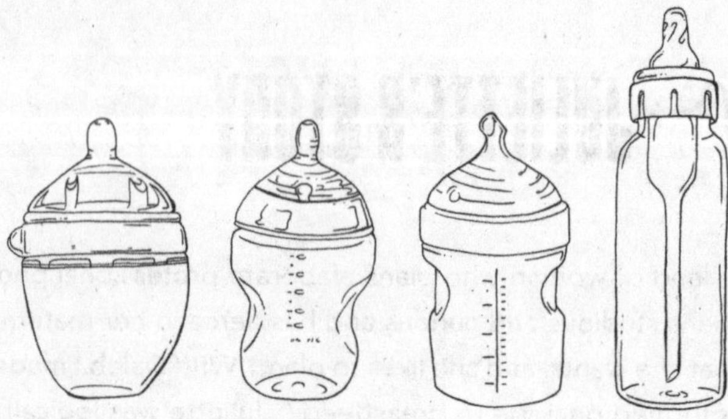

STORAGE SYSTEM BOTTLES

Some bottles are designed to integrate with pumping bags. While these streamline storage for some families, they are difficult to maneuver and use to pace feedings. I would start out with a more traditional bottle and acquire a system like this later when you know it will work well for you.

VENTS

Some bottles have vents to "prevent colic," the excessive crying that happens with some babies (see page 221). This is a bold claim, as the causes of colic are a bit of a mystery, but the vents slow the flow rate and can help a baby drink consistently without being flooded with milk and without swallowing air, which might cause an upset stomach. Any bottle given slowly and paced well can do this. The vents work well, but do add a lot of extra parts to clean.

SLOW-FLOW NIPPLES

All bottles are available with an assortment of nipple sizes. The size rating on a bottle nipple refers to the flow resistance on the milk. Think of this like resistance on a stationary bike or a weight-lifting machine. "Slow flow" is the highest resistance, and we want high resistance so that a baby has to work to develop their suck. There is generally no need to change this resistance over the course of bottle feeding unless suggested by a lactation professional or pediatrician. If your baby is over four months and seems very frustrated with the bottle, you can try adjusting the nipple to a higher flow rate (like a number 2, which is a medium-flow nipple). Some of these holes are manufactured by a machine puncturing the nipple. Dr. Brown's bottles are formed silicone and have the most standard flow rate.[15] This is irrelevant to most babies, but if you are an engineering nerd, these bottles are very precise tools.

BOTTLE MATERIALS

Plastic is lightweight, conducts temperature well, and is transparent. This makes it the most popular option. Some parents, however, have concerns about chemical leaching. While most bottles are now made with BPA-free plastics, some parents still prefer not to use them. They also discolor in the dishwasher.

Silicone is less porous than plastic and does not leach. It is less conductive than traditional plastic but still cools and warms well. The main drawback is that silicon is squishy, which makes it hard to standardize flow rate while holding a bottle in your hand.

Glass bottles are becoming more and more common. Some come with a silicon sleeve to prevent breakage and slipping. They are heavy, which is a consideration with grip strength. The main drawback to glass is that it insulates so well. It can take a long time to heat up or cool down milk in glass bottles. They are dishwasher safe, easiest to clean, and will last generations if you want. The other challenge of glass bottles is that they are not allowed at some daycares, so you need to check with your daycare about their policy.

Stainless steel is nonleaching and nonbreakable. It conducts temperature well, but it is opaque. This can make it very difficult to know how much liquid is in it and how much milk a baby has left.

PREPARING FORMULA

PREMIXED VS. POWDER

Infant formula comes in two forms.

Premixed

Ready to go, these bottles are shelf stable until you open them. They are much more expensive than powdered formula. These may be good to have in an emergency-preparedness kit or on road trips. Note that all premixed formula is not sterile. If your baby needs sterile formula for medical reasons, make sure the bottle says sterile.

HOW TO PREPARE PREMIXED FORMULA

1. Wash your hands.
2. Pour desired amount of premixed formula in bottle.
3. To warm the bottle, heat up a few ounces of water in a microwave or kettle and place in a mug. Place the bottle in the water for a few minutes. Remove bottle, swirl the formula and test for temperature on your wrist. It should feel warm, not hot.
4. Discard whatever was in the baby's bottle after feeding or within 2 hours.

Powder

Not sterile. You mix it with water to reconstitute it. It's extremely convenient, but you do need clean water.

HOW TO PREP POWDER FORMULA

1. Wash hands.
2. Fill bottle with desired amount of warm or room-temperature water.
3. Add the number of scoops indicated on the packaging.
4. **Store scoop in designated place:** either store the scoop in the clip place on the lid of the can of formula or, if there is not a place for it, designate a clean place. Do not plop it back in the powder where you will have to dig around for it and touch powder with your hands.
5. Shake up bottle.
6. Discard after feeding or within 2 hours of mixing at room temperature if not used immediately.

Open premixed formula or formula you have mixed yourself can sit in the refrigerator for twenty-four hours. This means that you can mix a pitcher of formula to keep in the fridge for the day. Some premixed formulas can be in the fridge for longer. You should follow the directions on the packaging.

You do not need a fancy formula-mixing machine. Formula is instant, and those machines can be difficult to clean and trap bacteria. Instead, I recommend leaving a pitcher of water on the counter that is kept at room temperature and mixing bottles from this. You can use a filtering pitcher if there are concerns about your water or the fluoride content of your water is considered too high for babies. You can find out if your water is considered safe for formula preparation by calling your local health department.

WELL WATER

If you live on a well, you may need to filter your water. It is a good idea to have your water tested and cleared for infants before your baby is born. You can bypass this and instead just filter well water before using it to mix bottles.

MIXING BREAST MILK AND FORMULA TOGETHER

Adding formula to breast milk changes its shelf life. Once formula is added, you will need to use it within the recommended safe storage window for formula. If your baby is premature and needs formula added as fortifier, you should prepare smaller bottles to make sure they get finished. Any fortified milk your baby doesn't take will need to be tossed out. If your baby drinks both breast milk and formula bottles because of gaps in milk production, you can just offer those bottles separately. Pool milk to save up for a breast milk bottle and in the meantime offer bottles of formula until you have enough for a breast-milk bottle. This will keep you from having to toss out hard earned breast milk.

HOW TO WASH BOTTLES

1. Store used bottles in a large dry basin until you are ready to wash
2. When you are ready to wash use a bottle brush or sponge that is ONLY for washing bottles. Add hot water and dish soap to the basin and brush the fully disassembled bottle parts. If bottles have small holes or channels use a pipe cleaner (this usually comes with the bottles) to wash inside them.
3. Rinse with hot water and place on a clean dish towel covered with a paper towel to dry.
4. You can also fully disassemble bottles and place them in the top rack of your dishwasher.

HOW TO GIVE A BABY A BOTTLE

Eating is how babies develop their mouth, head, and face shape. Sucking helps brings jaws forward, un-cones heads, and builds a foundation for eating solids and speaking. When we slow down a bottle feeding, it improves digestion and satiety (knowing when you are full). Slower bottles also help babies avoid swallowing air, which can cause uncomfortable gas pains. Do me a favor: swallow. Right now, without drinking anything. Did you swallow air? No, you swallow saliva. We swallow air when we drink too quickly, not because there is air in the bottle. Don't worry that a baby sucking on a bottle nipple without milk flow will cause gas; it won't. Feeding too quickly will. To counteract this, it's beneficial to practice paced bottle feeding. Paced bottle feeding is a method of giving babies bottles where they have to draw milk toward themselves. This slower process improves digestion and strengthens baby's muscles.

Other benefits of paced bottle feeding

- Time to recognize hunger and fullness cues
- Eating appropriate volumes/avoiding overfeeding
- Mouth development
- Less upset stomach
- Easier time going back and forth to the breast if you are nursing.

HOW TO DO PACED BOTTLE FEEDING

There are two goals in paced bottle feeding: the baby does the work, and the baby eats slowly. A paced bottle feed should take at least ten minutes. This kind of feeding reduces flow preference (if you are nursing and bottle feeding), builds sucking skills and oral strength, and helps babies learn their satiety cues.

A paced bottle is almost always parallel to the ground, so that instead of pouring milk into a baby's mouth, the baby is working to draw the milk out.

Start by setting yourself up somewhere comfortable. Somewhere with back support and pillows to stack on your lap. Then either sit baby up on your lap or lay them down on their side.

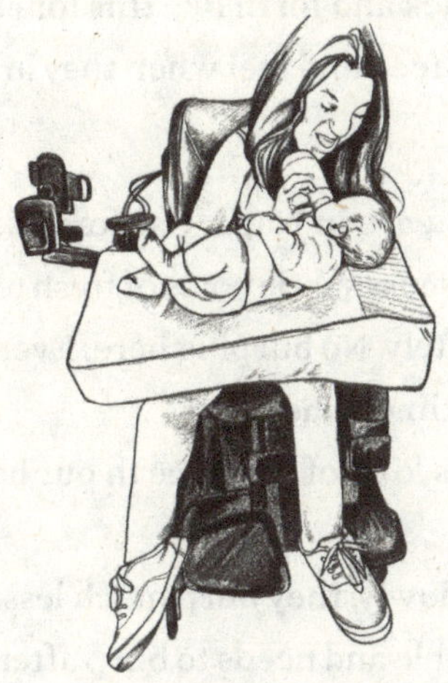

Hold the bottle in your hand like a pencil and tickle your baby's upper lip. Wait for them to do a big open mouth and then put the bottle nipple in their mouth to latch them onto the bottle. You want their mouth to be very open and full of bottle nipple. This is why I like narrow-necked bottles; I find they are easier to get a good latch. On a narrow-neck bottle, your baby's lips should be at or nearly at the collar of the bottle.

Wait for your baby to engage a solid suck and then tip the bottle toward them just enough that milk goes into the nipple. Then pull back ever so slightly on the bottle like you are playing a game of tug-of-war you want them to win.

If your baby is eating very quickly, you can tip the bottle back so milk pools back in the bottle and make them take a break. They will not swallow air. We swallow air when we drink too fast. They will just suck on the bottle nipple like a pacifier. After a minute or two, you can tip the bottle back to

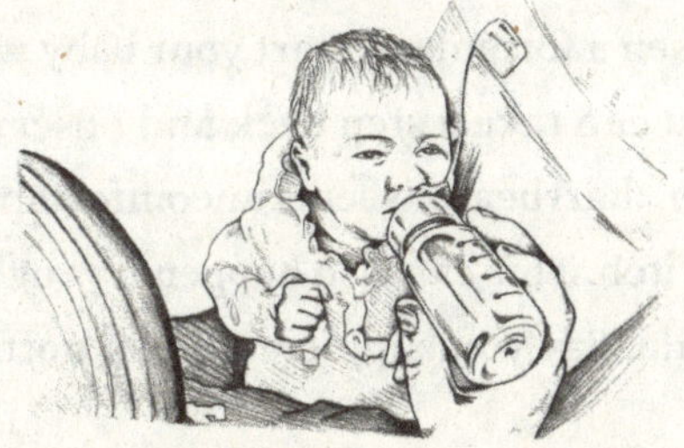

fill the nipple. Rocking back and forth like this for about ten minutes will help your baby pace their feed and feel when they are full.

BURPING AND GAS

Imagine you are in Napa, California, sipping wine, taking breaks to discuss subtle notes of fresh tennis ball can and oak, sipping politely. No burping here. Even if you are drinking a lovely sparkling wine.

We want to inspire this kind of elegance in our babies. Wine. Not beer funnel.

When we feed babies slowly, they burp much less.

If a baby is uncomfortable and needs to burp after most feedings, I will try to chase down a cause for this gas, but in the meantime, burping is a good skill to have.

Burping is done by pressure on the tummy, not the pats on the back. You can use the baby sit-ups technique on page 195. Place your baby on your lap so that the heel of your hand is below their ribs and their face is cradled in the web between your thumb and pointer. Leaning your baby forward, pat your baby's back like you are playing a hand drum. Some people like the classic look of an over-the-shoulder burp; that's fine, just make sure your baby is high enough on your shoulder that your shoulder is touching their stomach. You may also want to put a cloth down so you don't have to change your whole outfit if they spit up down your back.

TROUBLESHOOTING

WHEN TO SWITCH FORMULA

Switching formulas for upset stomachs

Once you have chosen a formula to start your baby with and have gotten a few weeks in, you can take a step back and observe. If your baby has rashes, constipation, diarrhea, or seems uncomfortable, it might be worth
rmula switch. This can also happen if your baby abruptly starts
re formula. Say you supplemented a bottle or two a day, but

ARSALAN'S STORY

"Both of our daughters had difficulty with feeding in their first few months after birth. We were particularly flummoxed with our elder daughter, as we had no experience or knowledge about what to do." They met with a lactation consultant, who taught them paced bottle feeding and completely changed their approach. "It was a moment of profound relief after our first session. I still remember that day vividly, the aha moment when I learned how to do paced bottle feeding and saw it work!"

Arsalan felt more bonded by paying close attention to these slower and more deliberate bottles. "Looking back, those are such precious memories, and I will never forget the cuddles! When our younger daughter joined us, all of the technical skills to effectively do paced bottle feeding came rushing back and significantly reduced our anxiety during those early days. I can safely say that if we had not learned this technique with the most patient of teachers, we would've been so overwhelmed and defeated."

went all-formula when you returned to work. This change in the amount of formula your baby is getting may reveal a sensitivity that warrants a change.

Start with the most likely culprits. In the listing of ingredients on the back of the formula, you will notice about ten ingredients and then the words "less than 2%." The ingredients before that marker make up the majority of the formula and are most likely to be causing the issue. (For more on formula and what's in it, refer to page 77.)

If your baby has an upset stomach, irritated skin, or a lot of gas, start by looking at the protein in your baby's formula.

Proteins

When we digest proteins, we use enzymes to break them into smaller pieces that we can absorb. These smaller pieces are called peptides. Cow's milk has larger proteins than breast milk which means that they need more enzymes and time to get chopped up enough for your baby to digest them. This is called hydrolysis. While our adult nutrition knowledge might lead us to want a formula that is less processed, you can think of it as the opposite for babies: the more processed the formula- the less work your baby has to do to digest it. That can make some babies more comfortable.

A formula that has these smaller broken-down proteins will have "partially hydrolyzed" in front of some of the proteins in that first few ingredients. These formulas can be especially good for babies with eczema as that is a sign of a systemic digestion issue.

Some babies need those proteins chopped up even smaller to make the formula even easier to digest. These are fully hydrolyzed formulas and you will see those words in the ingredients. These are also known as hypoallergenic formulas because the proteins are so small that even a baby who is allergic to milk can digest them because they have been so broken down from the original cow's milk source. These formulas are pretty stinky and very expensive. They are life-saving and important for babies who need them, but unless they are recommended by your doctor: stick to a partially hydrolyzed option.

LOOK AT THE CASEIN-TO-WHEY RATIO

Another change we have to make to cow's milk to make it suitable nutrition for human newborns is adjusting the ratio of whey to casein. Whey and casein are two categories of protein (like curds and whey). Human milk has more whey than casein. If your baby is constipated or having other symptoms of an upset stomach, try switching to a formula that has whey added to it and see if the issues resolve. Look for whey to be specifically listed in the first set of ingredients.

Carbohydrates

The next possible culprit of an upset stomach could be the carbohydrate.

The main carbohydrate in human milk is lactose. That's why I recommend that families start with a lactose-based formula, unless their baby is preterm. Preterm babies do not yet make enough lactase (the enzyme that breaks down lactose) to digest it well. Some term babies also just don't do as well on a fully lactose formula. Try gradually moving them onto a formula with a lower lactose ratio and a higher ratio of other carbohydrates to see how they do.

Fats

The least likely cause of tummy trouble is the fat source. It does happen, though. Human milk contains palmitic acid, an amino acid that is similar to palm oil but has some key differences on the molecule. This can create digestion issues in some babies and specifically presents with constipation. If your baby is constipated and changing the proteins and carbohydrate sources didn't help, consider shifting the fat source to one with less or no palm oil.

HOW TO SWITCH FORMULAS

Once you've identified a new formula that you think will be a better fit for your baby based on symptoms, you can start gradually switching. A good baseline is to switch by one quarter per day. If your baby gets diarrhea or has more digestive issues, you can go slower. If your baby is having severe symptoms on their current formula (blood in stool or other allergic symptoms) touch base with your pediatrician for monitoring and switch directly to the new formula.

Day 1: ¾ old formula, ¼ new formula

Day 2: ½ old formula, ½ new formula

Day 3: ¼ old formula, ¾ new formula

Day 4: all new formula, stay there for at least two weeks before switching, unless you see severe symptoms (blood in stool, allergic reaction, etc., in which case you should call your pediatrician).

If this mixing math is tricky (what is three quarters of a three-ounce bottle?!), then you can mix a pitcher of the correct ratio for the day and keep it in the fridge. Pour out a bottle of the desired amount and warm it in a mug of hot water or bottle warmer.

If your baby has some weird symptoms, like a change in sleep, an uptick in symptoms, etc., stay at that ratio for a day or two to rule out if it was coincidence or caused by the switch. If you are having trouble finding a formula that works well for your baby, I recommend consulting the work of Dr. Bridget Young and her website, babyformulaexpert.com. She consulted with me for all of the formula information in this book and is a brilliant researcher and problem solver. She offers great advice to help families navigate formula feeding.

CHAPTER 7

PUMPING AND EXPRESSING

Whether you are pumping to bottle feed without nursing (exclusively pumping) or pumping in addition to nursing to have milk for another caregiver to give your baby, pumping is a hallmark of modern feeding. Pumps are a relatively new technology, and I am elated that the technology seems to improve every day. This tool is both a source of freedom and a prison. It allows us to keep our bodies safe and comfortable and provide milk while being away from our babies. It can also create the expectation that we must provide in this way for our babies. Remember, you get to choose how you use this tool and if and when it works for you.

Some people find that nursing isn't for them or isn't working, but still want to provide their own milk. If you go this route, respect the hard work you are doing and continually assess if it is working for you and ask for help in other areas of life and baby care to make time for pumping.

As pump technology has improved, pumps have become more comfortable and more portable (I once saw a woman pumping at the bar with friends, and she is my hero—see page 70 for how to calculate alcohol in breast milk). Just like with nursing, it takes some time to find your groove with pumping. Finding your right suction, flange size, and timing is all a learning experience. Once that is all dialed in, it should not be painful, but most people feel like it is a chore.

You will want a hospital-grade pump (see page 40 for advice on how to choose) and good pumping bra, and you may want an on-the-go option if there is a portable pump that meets your budget and needs.

MARCI'S STORY

Marci has fed kids pretty much every way possible with her three children: Jackson, Eliza and Penelope. She has exclusively pumped; she has exclusively formula fed; she has exclusively nursed. She has tube fed, and she has mixed and matched. Marci, whose eldest son has Down Syndrome, is an absolute expert at changing plans. She exclusively pumped for her first, who was tube fed for nine months due to his prematurity and disability. "We lived five minutes from the hospital, and they loaned us the same pump for home that they had in the NICU." She pumped every two hours for weeks and weeks building up a huge reserve while her baby grew and got ready to eat. "I wouldn't have been able to do it without seven months of leave, but for me, it worked."

When she had her second child, she figured she would see if she had missed out on anything by pumping and tube feeding. "I just remember us both crying all the time." Eliza was so fussy that her doctor suggested cutting dairy and eventually trying hypoallergenic formula. "She was four months old, and the change was NIGHT AND DAY within twenty-four hours." Marci donated her stash, pumped for a few more weeks as she weaned down her milk production to dry up, and switched to formula feeding.

The gift of being an experienced parent is an intimate understanding of your options and what matters to you and what doesn't. "I remembered how the screaming and pain impacted my mental health with Eliza and said: *You know what, I'll just pump.*" With American shelves nearly devoid of formula in 2022 due to a manufacturer recall, formula feeding wasn't a stable option. "I latched Penelope for about the first forty-eight hours and fed her a few syringes of colostrum I had hand expressed in pregnancy." Then, she pumped. "I'm going to pump through the winter, when she's six months old, then use up what's in the freezer; it's just so much more convenient to pump." Marci pumps every two hours during the day while juggling her older two kids' schedules and waits three to four hours between pumping at night.

"I didn't feel any more bonded from nursing Eliza than tube feeding Jackson, so I just know pumping for Penelope is the right choice this time."

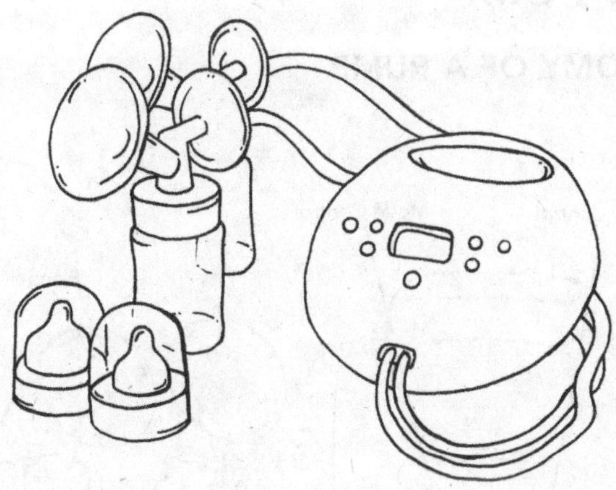

A NOTE ON EXCLUSIVE PUMPING

On page 236, you'll find more information about understanding your body's storage capacity, this will help you navigate how often you need to pump after the six-week mark. Before six weeks, you will want to express eight to twelve times per day to set a good level of production. As long as you have pump some of these during the night, when your brain is most hormonally receptive, you can cluster some pumps to times when you have more help or when your baby is best regulated without being held, or to give yourself some big chunks of sleep. Exclusive pumping is extremely hard work; you will need rest and support to make it possible.

Use hand expression as a tool to support pumping. This will keep your production up and help in the event of pump-malfunction emergencies. A good support system is also key. There are some amazing experts in exclusive pumping online. They can offer tools and community. I find that these individuals are the experts on pump technology, which seems to change every day. Use them to help find effective and portable options that allow you to live your life and still express milk.

HOW TO PUMP

THE ANATOMY OF A PUMP

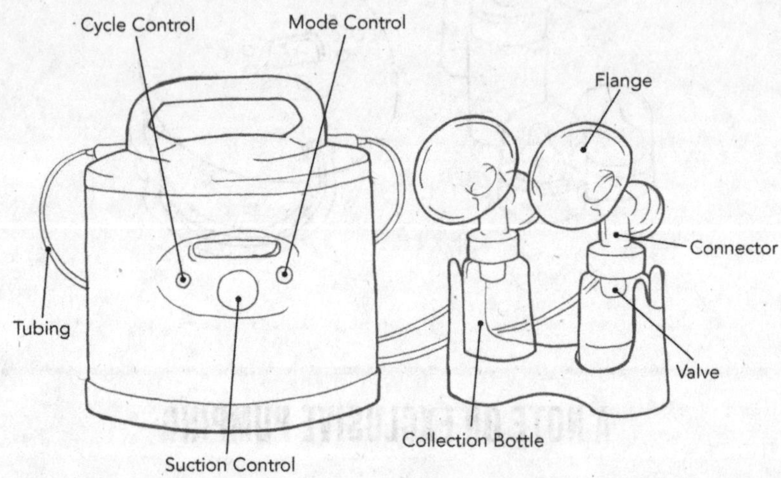

Flange. This is where the pump makes contact with your body. This part needs to fit your nipples well and be lubricated. Your flanges should be cleaned regularly.

Valve. The valve creates the vacuum that draws milk out so it can collect in the bottles. These parts also need to be cleaned regularly. If they have any rips or holes, your pump won't suck.

Tubing. The tubing moves air from the pump to the flange. It doesn't actually touch milk, so it should not be washed. If you do wash them, it's hard to get the water out again, which could lead to mold—gross!—so they should stay dry.

Controls. This part tells the pump to mimic a baby's suck, which tells your brain to release the hormones to make milk.

Most pumps have three controls: cycle (how many times a pump sucks in a minute, a.k.a. speed), suction (how hard it sucks), and mode (a button that goes from fast little sucks used to trigger a letdown into big slow sucks to move milk).

These controls should be adjusted so that they work for you each pumping session, following a basic sucking pattern of fast/light then slow/strong. The amount of suction should feel comfortable but effective. Pumping shouldn't hurt. Just like with nursing, pain is a sign to get help.

Collection bottles. These bottles come with your pump and are just a place to collect milk. You may or may not use these bottles to feed your baby. You can use adapters to switch them to pump directly into storage bags or a different kind of bottle.

Connector. This piece of plastic connects the flanges to the valve and collection bottle. It is the intersection that brings all of the functional pieces together.

SETTING UP YOUR PUMP

Flange fit

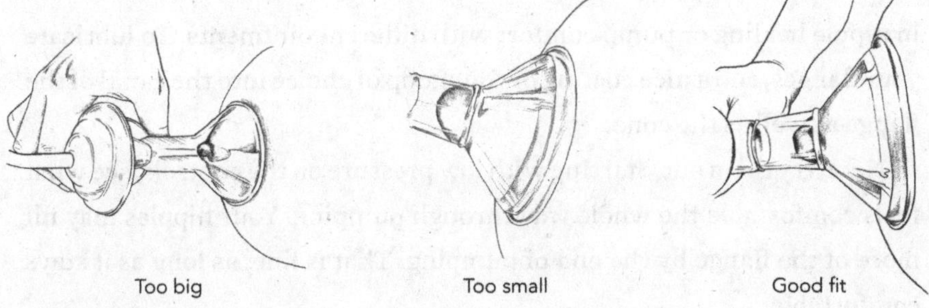

Pumps often come with one size of flange. This is ridiculous because nipples come in many, many shapes and sizes. Your nipples are like Goldilocks, so make the extra effort to find a set of flanges that are just right. Nipples are also often different from the beginning of a pumping session to the end of one, and what is comfortable sometimes changes from day to day. Flanges are easy to wash, and there are many great aftermarket and manufacturer-made options. Once you get started pumping, take a look at your options, and maybe ask friends if you can have the flanges they have ruled out as definitely not working for them.

Also, remember that you have two nipples. They may have different needs.

To find the right fit, hold the flanges onto your nipples without attaching them to the pump. Your nipple should fill the center with an eighth of an inch or so around it. Breast tissue should not be pulled into the flange along with the nipple.

Once you have found a good size, prepare to give it a try and realize that it may take a few trials to find your just-right flange. The most important thing is comfort. If milk is flowing and you aren't in pain while pumping or after, who cares what it looks like?

Lubricate

I cannot stress this enough. Pumping is your body coming into contact with plastic over and over and over again for fifteen-plus minutes. You can use your nipple cream, household oils like olive oil or coconut oil, shea butter, or moisturizer like Vaseline. Goop is goop. People usually have a preference for what they like to use, but there isn't a documentable difference in nipple healing or pump comfort with different ointments. To lubricate your flanges, rub a nice coating of your goop of choice into the canal of the flange as well as the cone.

Next, try them out. Starting with low pressure on the controls, see what feels comfortable the whole way through pumping. Your nipples may fill more of the flange by the end of pumping. That is fine, as long as it stays comfortable.

Some people's nipples are very elastic and fill whatever flange they come into contact with. Find your most comfortable fit and then assess whether pumping is right for you. You may find that hand expression, formula, or donor milk is a better option than putting your body through stress for a system that wasn't designed for you.

Pump settings

Pumps come with increasingly varied settings. The two main ones mimic the beginning of a baby's feeding: fast letdown suck and the big slow milk-moving suck (unlike a baby, pumps don't have little comfort sucks, because you do not need to comfort your pump). Both should feel comfortable, and you can cycle through them to meet your needs. The letdown mode (it may have a different name based on your pump) has fast, lighter sucks. The milk-moving mode does slower, stronger sucks.

Many people use the letdown mode, then switch to the milk-moving mode once they see milk flowing. Know that you can cycle back through the letdown mode any time milk flow slows down and you want to get things moving again.

PUMPING TO BUILD UP A MILK STASH

Something about our culture of scarcity, pressure to breastfeed, and productivity culture has resulted in a full-on obsession with one's milk stash. I have seen deep freezers full; I have seen the panic over the one lone bag in the freezer. The reality is, milk is a renewable resource and store-bought formula is fine. The goal when pumping and freezing milk is to feel calm and secure about it. You are not defined by your milk stash and milk stashes are not infallible. One power outage, new food allergy, or discovery of high lipase can render gallons of pumped milk unusable. This milk represents your time. Time when you could have been sleeping, showering, or hanging out with your kid. Try to find out how much you need to feel comfortably secure and then don't overdo it. Leave the freezer for what it was meant for: ice cream and things to put in the oven when you are too lazy to make dinner. (See page 279 for a guide to how much milk to stash.)

ADDING PUMPING FOR EXCLUSIVE NURSERS

If nursing has been going great and there is no need to pump or offer bottles, carry on for the first two weeks. It is great to master one system before adding another variable. At two to four weeks, there is a good developmental window in which to introduce bottles. This can be done via formula or donor milk (see supplementation page 213) or by starting to pump. Since the goal here isn't supplementing your baby's diet, just getting them accustomed to bottles, there is no need to worry about volumes of pumping. I find that the midmorning pump is a great place to start.

GETTING STARTED

If you are nursing, identify your "first morning feeding." This is the one before you get up and have some breakfast and a brew. Nurse just as you normally do.

Settle your baby into a nap/arms of another caregiver/bouncer/floor mat.

Gather whatever you need (coffee, water bottle, remote, snack, pump, and pump parts).

Starting with your pump set to the lowest setting, attach your pump and engage the fast suck mode (this is different on different pumps: some start here; some you need to press a button to engage it). Gradually bring the suction up to where it is comfortable, but you are able to feel it.

Once you see milk flow, you can engage the slower suction (again, this will vary from pump to pump). Adjust your suction. Let the machine do its thing, doing some massage if you feel like it, for about ten to twenty minutes, or until you see milk flow significantly slow down.

Congratulations, you pumped!

You may want to begin to integrate this into your morning routine to create bottles for other caregivers to pitch in at other parts of the day or to put in storage. Alternately, you can do this a few times a week to work on bottle skills. See page 202 on how to introduce bottles.

PUMPING TROUBLESHOOTING

Pumping is its own whole world, but many of the complications are the same as those encountered in nursing: mastitis (page 128), sore or damaged nipples, plugged ducts (page 125). As for the pump itself, pumping ranges a lot pump to pump. There are so many ways to configure different parts and motors that it's easy to get a bit lost. Remember that some pumps, such as in-bra continuous suction pumps, require a different flange fit from conventional pumps. If you are having a sudden drop in pumping output, it is a good idea to do a pumping audit:

- Take everything apart and give it a good cleaning and inspection.
- Are the valves intact and free of fat buildup?
- Are there any tears or punctures along the tubing?
- Is the attachment to the pump itself snug?

PASSIVE COLLECTION

Some people leak. If you don't, don't worry about it. It doesn't mean anything, just skip this section and move on. If you do, we may as well take advantage.

There are two kinds of passive-collection devices: the kind you tuck in your bra and the kind that uses suction and dangle. If you are collecting while nursing, you'll want to treat that milk like milk you pumped and use or store milk within six to eight hours, and wash your hand pump at that point, as well.

With an in-bra collection system between feeding, you should process that milk every hour or so and use it or move it into storage. Bacteria grows much faster at high temperatures (like 98.6 F), so it can spoil faster than if it were on the counter (assuming your house is between 60 and 75 degrees).

Passive collection is also a great way to take the pressure off when you are uncomfortably full. If you have high production and are full more often than your baby eats, this is a great way to get comfortable when your baby only needs to nurse on one side (page 133).

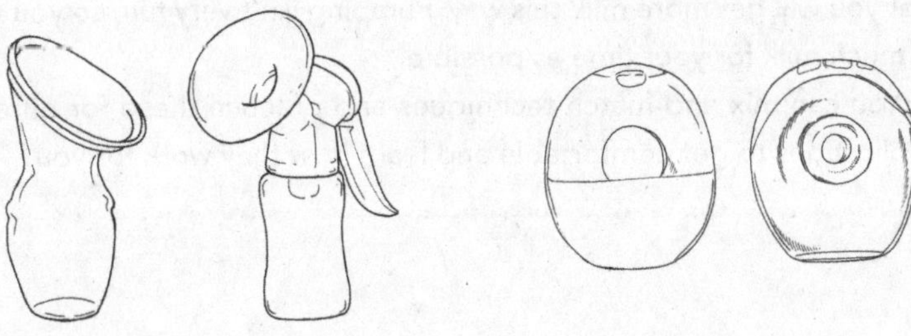

HAND EXPRESSION

Next up on the milk-removal menu is hand expression. I know, I know, this one feels frustratingly slow and confusing to most of us, but I promise that it is an important tool to have in your tool kit. Hand expression is essential for emergencies to keep your body healthy if you are away from your baby and pump. It makes pumping more efficient, and for some people is actually more efficient and "enjoyable" than pumping. Or at least less annoying with less stuff to wash. Do you own a food processor? It's great, right? It can chop three pounds of carrots so well! But can we all agree that lugging it out of the cabinet, putting it together, and then washing all the parts isn't entirely worth it to chop half an onion? Some basic knife skills are also a good thing to have.

You may be tempted to skip this section, as hand expressing couldn't possibly be as effective as your fancy pump. Truth is, for some people it is much more effective, and these two systems can be used in concert. Hand expression can usually get a letdown going faster than the letdown mode on your pump. It is also better at fully softening your chest at the end of a pumping session to keep production up and help you avoid or address plugged ducts.

MORE EFFECTIVE PUMPING

When babies nurse, they use both suction and compression. Pumps only use suction. So, if you pump without any hand expression techniques, you are missing half of the milk-expression puzzle. Most people find it easier to get milk flowing with compression than suction and research shows that you will get more milk this way. Pumping isn't very fun, so you want as much milk for your time as possible.

You can mix and match techniques and practice these for different applications to get comfortable and learn how they work for you.

Getting started: What you'll need

A cloth. Hand expression is messy until you get the hang of it. A cloth to wipe up drips or tuck into your clothes is good to have on hand.

Oil. Coconut oil and olive oil both work great. Barely any will get in the milk, but hands sliding against your skin will be more comfortable and efficient.

A big bowl. Aim is tricky with the multidirectional outlets of a nipple. A big bowl on a table or in your lap is the best way to catch all the directions without worrying about it. A clean salad or popcorn bowl will do the trick. If you love hand expression, you can then upgrade to some great, uniquely shaped collection vessels, but start with a bowl.

Getting the milk out[16]

These strategies are for moving milk, either to fill a spoon for spoon feeding, to get relief when you are out without a pump or baby, while pumping, or for collection. I learned these from the brilliant Francie Webb, who went on a *Eat, Pray, Love*–style journey into self-acceptance through hand expression. If these techniques and hand expression in general are working for you, check our her book *Go Milk Yourself.*

THE C-CLAMP

Making a large C-shape with your hands, hold your breast and push the C-shape directly into your chest wall, then squeeze your fingers together. Out, in, together, out, in, together.

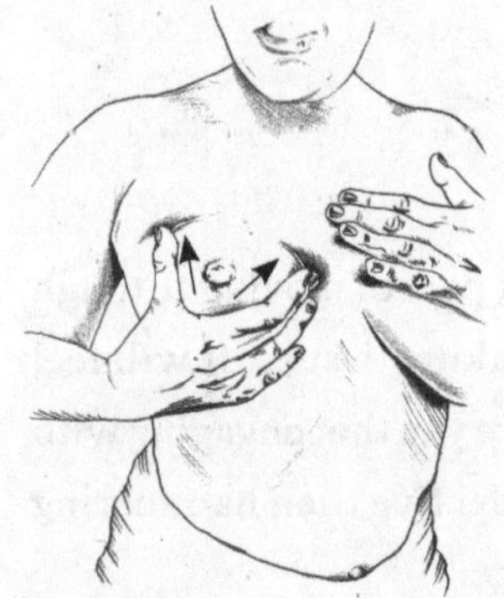

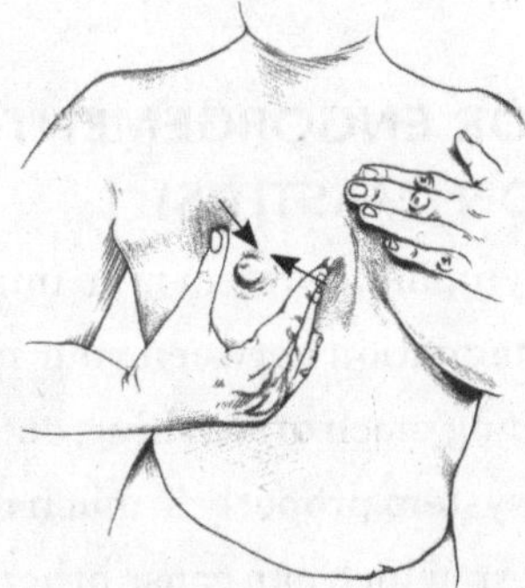

SCRAPE THE BROWNIE BATTER

With the back of your hand, slowly slide against your breast from the outside toward the nipple, work your way around your breast, slowly pressing toward the nipple when you have flow. Just as with brownie batter in a bowl, make sure you didn't miss any spots.

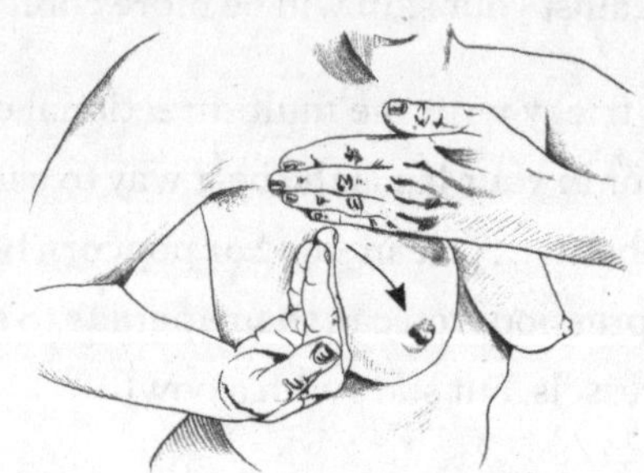

FINGERPRINTING

Make your C-shape with your thumb near the edge of your areola, then roll your thumb toward your nipple like you are fingerprinting your thumb. Do this until flow slows, then rotate to another angle and fingerprint again.

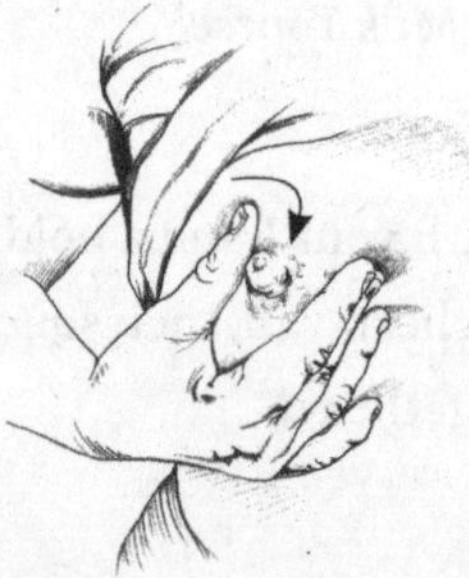

MASSAGE FOR ENGORGEMENT OR INFECTION (MASTITIS)

Engaging your lymphatic system is an important part of moving through these kinds of stagnation between your milk-making tissues. It will feel like you aren't doing much of anything, but I assure you that engaging with your lymphatic system properly is much more effective than hammering away at your chest, which can cause other damage.

Small circles to engage the lymphatic system

With your pointer finger, gently rub ten little circles above your collar bone at the base of your neck. About where a necklace chain hits. No need to press too hard; you are just saying, "Hello, wake up."

Repeat with ten small circles in the chub of your armpit.

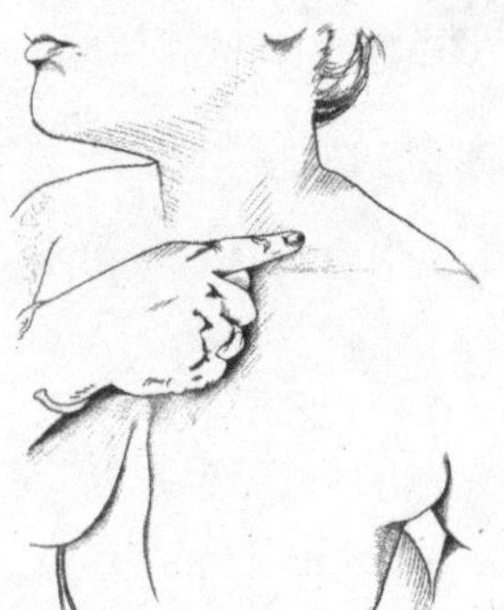

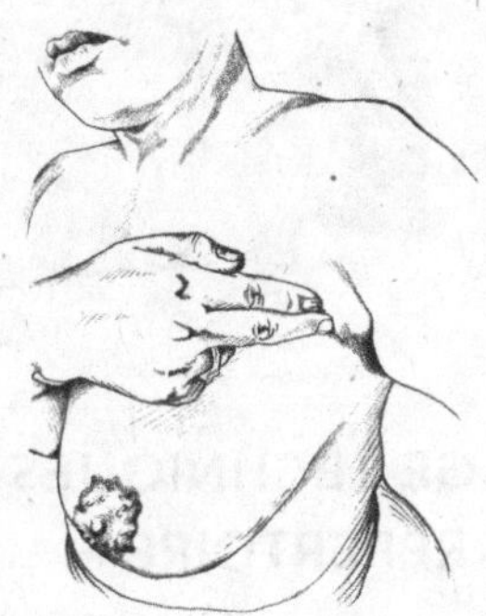

Press back

Push flat palms backward into your breast, straight toward your rib cage. Hold your hand there with firm pressure and count to thirty. (BONUS: This will stop an embarrassing unexpected letdown. Just cross your arms across your chest and press in for thirty seconds in a meeting, for instance.)

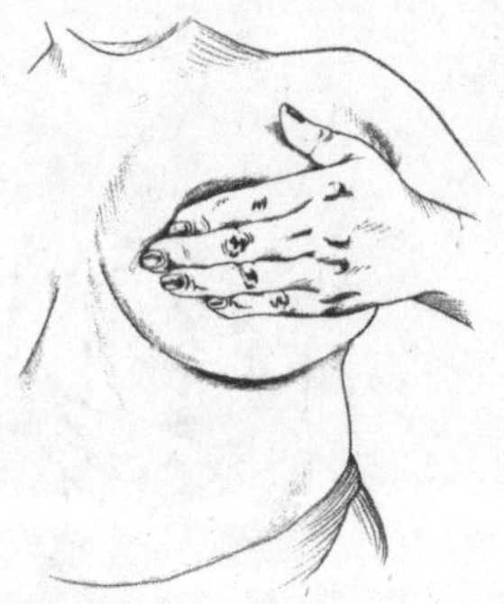

Lift up

Lean back or lie as flat as you can. Using both hands, find the edges of your breast tissue and lift your breast straight up to the ceiling up off your chest wall. Count to thirty, repeat on the other side.

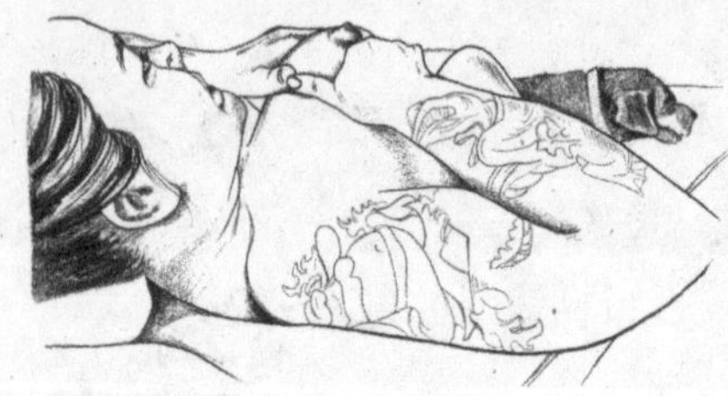

OTHER MASSAGE TECHNIQUES TO KEEP IN YOUR REPERTOIRE

These techniques to evert nipples, reduce swelling around clogs, and stay comfortable between feedings are good to learn while you are learning hand expression.

Shake it up

Hold your breast in your palm, two palms if you have large breasts, and shake your breast up and down. Sing the chorus of Taylor Swift's "Shake It Off" to yourself.

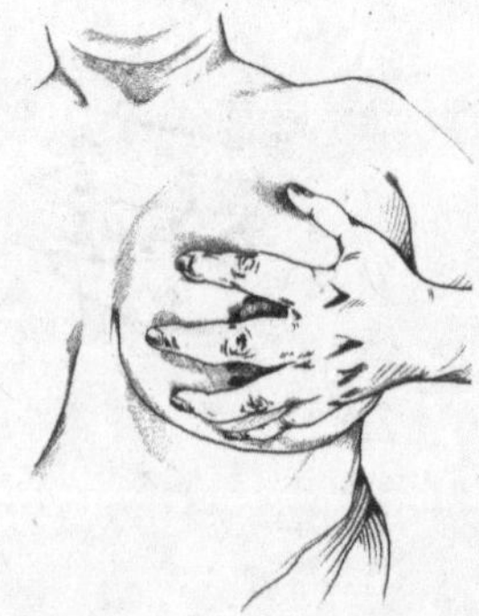

Citrus twist

Placing one palm on the top of your breast and one on the bottom, twist like you are juicing and orange, or opening a bank vault. Flip your hands and go the other direction.

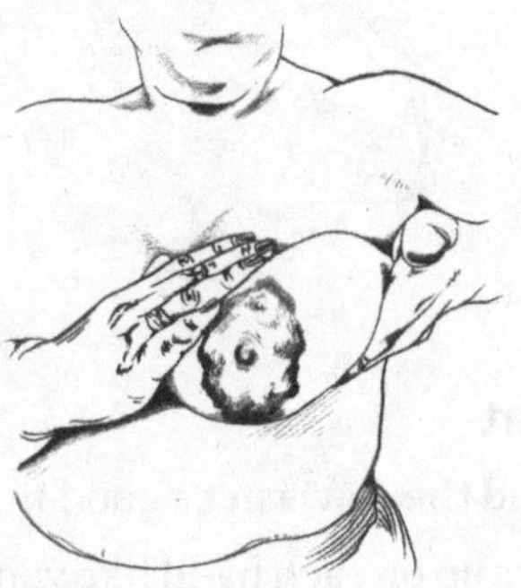

Up and out

Using the sides of your hands or four fingertips together, make big sweeping motions from your nipple to your armpit. Working in sections, do this for all 360 degrees of your breast. You are moving fluid up toward your lymphatic system so it can drain away.

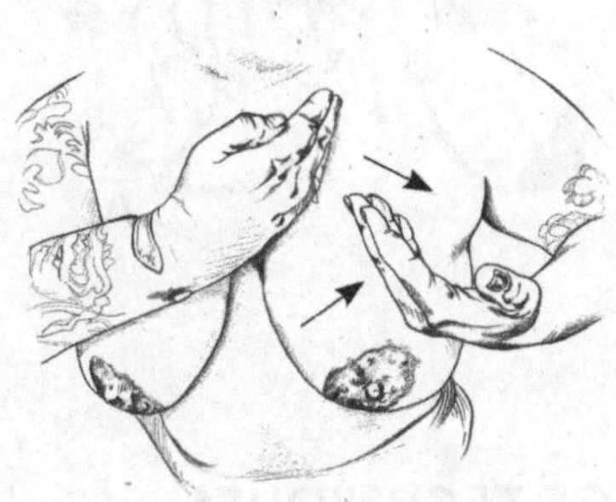

NIPPLE EVERSION

If your chest is uncomfortably full/so full that it is hard to latch (this is especially common the first week of nursing as milk transitions, or first thing in the morning), these techniques can help you get your nipple everted enough to get things moving.

The Claw

With your fingers facing you, make a claw by bending your fingertips toward each other. Push that claw firmly into your breast around your nipple, hold it there, and count to thirty.

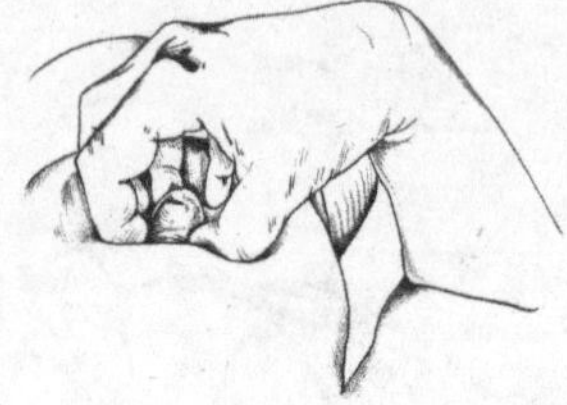

The Flight Attendant

If you have long nails and the claw isn't a good fit, try the Flight Attendant instead. Hold two fingers up on each hand like you are directing passengers to the exit rows on an airplane. Press your fingers flat against your breast on either side of your nipple, parallel to one another, pointing to your toes. Then go the other direction so each set of fingers is pointing at the opposite armpit. Hold each direction firmly for thirty seconds.

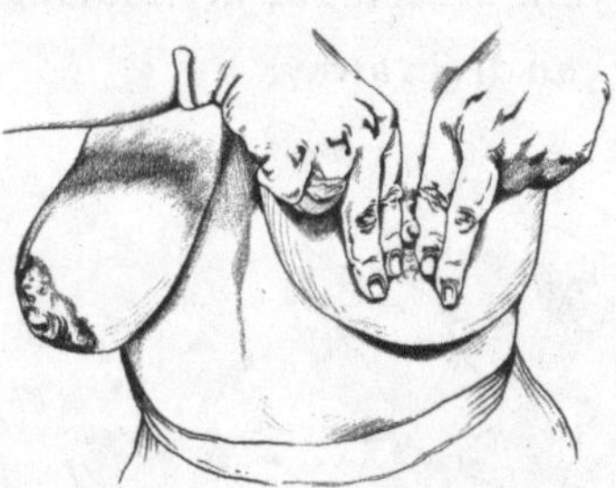

UNPLUG MASSAGE TECHNIQUES

Plugged ducts happen, and they are terrible. They can feel like a little ball or a concerning knot in your breast. They can lead to mastitis and are just downright uncomfortable. Use all of these strategies to move them. People often bruise themselves trying to move a plug. Try to be nice to yourself. Oxytocin gets things flowing, and pain blocks oxytocin.

Here are the additional hand expression techniques to use with that protocol. Remember this tissue is a gland, not a muscle. Be gentle. You aren't actually feeling the plug, you are feeling the swelling and fascia around the clogged duct. The goal is to ease the discomfort, not force milk out. (For more on mastitis, see page 128.)

STORING EXPRESSED MILK

You will hear and see a wide range of milk storage guidelines. I chose to operate based on Academy of Breastfeeding Medicine's guideline. They change their recommendations from time to time, so if you are googling milk storage, start there. The recommendations at time of publication are: human milk is super safe at room temperature (60 degrees–85 degrees F) for four hours. It is also safe up go eight hours in "very clean conditions." It is fine in the refrigerator for four days, but up to eight. It is optimal to use milk after six months in the freezer, but it is acceptable up to twelve.[17]

There is some variability in these recommendations. That is because your room temperature in January in Iowa and my room temperature in August in North Carolina can have a big variability in temperature. You may also have less tolerance for risk in this area, or your baby may be immune-compromised in a way that leaves no wiggle room.

The goal is to approach milk storage as safe food prep. Wash your hands before expressing and handing milk. Store used bottles and pump parts in a dry basin (not your sink) and fill with hot soapy water when you are washing them. Dry them on a clean dish cloth with a paper towel over it. While this is not surgery and thus not sterile, cleanliness means less bacteria to bloom at room temperature.

When in doubt, smell it.

Milk of any kind gives off a sour smell when it has spoiled. If you think it has been too warm too long: sniff your milk. If it smells spoiled—toss it.

A FEW HACKS BASED ON HUMAN MILK'S LONG SHELF LIFE

Pooling milk. You can pool milk that you have pumped. Some people keep a jar or thermos in their fridge and add to it as they pump. Then they make bottles from that pooled milk. At the end of each day if there is milk left over, pour it into separate bottles for the next day or freeze any excess. Wash your container and begin again.

If you are pumping and bottle feeding at night: You can keep everything on your night stand and wait until the morning to wash everything. It is safe to reuse your pump parts. You can also make a bottle for the first feeding of the night and set it on your night stand. Then when you pump, that becomes the next bottle which can also sit at room temperature on your night stand.

Using an unfinished bottle: For term, healthy babies, it is safe to feed them the remainder of an unfurnished bottle at the next feeding. Do not, however, add new milk to this bottle. Finish the one from the last feeding and then start fresh with a new smaller bottle if your baby is still hungry.

Frozen milk between six months and a year: You'll notice that using milk within six months is "optimal" and up to a year is "acceptable." This is because at the temperature of regular household freezers there may be a decline in nutrients and bacteria fighting components. There isn't enough research to prove this one way or the other. This does not mean that it is spoiled or nutrient-less. It is just a decline from where it started.

Labeling stored milk: Milk storage bags have an area for labeling. This labeling system can go down to the minute you pumped it. I find this to be overkill. The date, or month is adequate to give you a sense of whether it is more than a year old and if it needs to be tossed.

High lipase: Lipase is an enzyme that starts breaking down milk as soon as it is expressed. This is great when babies are directly nursing, but over time in storage it creates a soapy taste. Some people's milk has more lipase and some babies are more sensitive to the taste of it. There is nothing wrong with this milk, it just doesn't taste the same. If your baby is refusing your stored milk due to high lipase you may just have to donate or toss it. If this is a known dynamic for you, you can prevent the lipase development by pooling your milk and then bringing it to a bare simmer on the stove: just until a few bubbles appear at the edges. Then let it cool and store as you normally do.

SECTION THREE

THE FIRST YEAR OF FEEDING.

CHAPTER 8

PREPARING TO GIVE BIRTH

There is a lot of talk about how people should and shouldn't give birth and how that impacts nursing. Beware of social pressures around "good" births and "bad" births. In reality, you have very little control over the kind of birth you have, so while the impacts birth has on feeding are important, you shouldn't confuse them with factors you can control. You are not a failure if birth or feeding don't go to plan. Additionally, birth interventions are tools. They are not traps; they are not inherently dangerous. People who need fewer tools in their birth are not better or more prepared than those who need every tool there is. If you are preparing for birth, try to learn about all of the tools rather than ignore them. Understanding a tool will not make you need it, but it can assist you in making decisions about how and when to use it.

A good example is epidurals. So-called natural or unmedicated birth is not better than births that require an epidural. Those parents are not tougher or more prepared. They simply had a birth that did not require that tool. Epidurals are a combination of pain medications that are injected into the epidural space of the spine. No two epidurals are the same, and no two reactions to epidurals are the same. Some babies born after an epidural will be a little dozier after birth while those drugs leave their system. That's normal; they will wake up and catch up on their eating skills within a few hours. Some birthing people may respond to an epidural in a way that makes feeding after birth more difficult; maybe you'll feel shaky and holding a baby might be challenging. This isn't a reason not to use an epidural; it is a reason to ask for help with feeding after having one. Ask for more pillows to support your baby and for someone else to help them latch while you rest.

HOW DIFFERENT BIRTH TYPES CAN IMPACT FEEDING

VACUUM-ASSISTED AND FORCEPS-ASSISTED BIRTH

These tools are used to get a baby out more quickly or adjust an angle of a baby in a poor position for birth. Babies who have been holding a less-than-ideal position in pregnancy or labor can have compression to the tiny nerves that help a baby suck. If you needed one of these tools, it's possible that your baby will need extra help with tummy time and massage to correct this nerve impingement and coordinate an effective suck (see baby alignment, page 53).

DEEP SUCTION AFTER BIRTH

Babies have a lot of mucus and amniotic fluid when they are born and sometimes need deep suction in their mouth right after birth to jumpstart breathing. This can make babies temporarily averse to stuff being put in their mouth, and they may need us to go more slowly with latch while they build a new association.

CESAREAN BIRTH

A surgical birth has a very different recovery from a vaginal one. They can both range from very difficult to very manageable. Having a large incision at your midsection can make getting comfortable while nursing difficult. Pain can impact how your milk flows, so you should absolutely use and keep up with the pain medications your doctor has prescribed. Additionally, milk transition (page 182) takes a bit longer after a cesarean birth.

IV FLUIDS IN LABOR

Intravenous (IV) fluids help people stay hydrated while giving birth. They can cause swelling at the extremities, which includes breasts. This can make engorgement when your milk transitions more intense (see page 115 for more on engorgement and how to reduce it). They can also impact a baby's birth weight. When a baby whose birth parent has had fluids is born, they also have more fluid in their bodies, which is completely safe and fine. They will simply pee it off soon after birth. We assume babies will lose up to 10 percent of their body weight in the first week after birth as milk transitions. Birth weight can be inflated by fluids in labor, making the 10 percent a less accurate measure of how your baby is doing with eating. You can ask for a weight check six to twelve hours after birth and use that to calculate weight loss after birth for a more accurate measurement.

HEMORRHAGE

The most common, and honestly, frightening birth complication is hemorrhage. When the placenta detaches, your body needs to quickly clot over a wound the size of a dinner plate. While some bleeding is normal, excessive bleeding is dangerous. Some people lose enough blood to come close to needing or to need a transfusion. This can cause fatigue, anaemia, and a delay to milk transition. Talk to your doctor about the specifics of your hemorrhage and how to best mitigate these symptoms and how to support your milk production. An iron supplement, transfusion, and a focus on hydration can help you recover more quickly and produce more milk if that is your goal. It also may just take time, and it is okay to supplement your baby while your body recovers.

LABOR-PAIN MANAGEMENT

Narcotic pain management (which includes epidurals) also impact babies. This is not dangerous, and is ideally used judiciously by providers. It can make babies sleepy after birth, which can make for lackadaisical nursers. Babies will become more alert and better able to eat within a few hours.

POSTPARTUM PAIN

Pain is very common after birth. Being in pain can impact letdown, milk production, bonding, and general wellbeing. Advocating for your pain management might be harder based on who you are. There is a lot of evidence that women as a whole, Black people, fat people, and people with chronic pain have a hard time being believed about pain and having it well-managed. Do what you can to speak up if you are in pain. Know that the pain meds given to birthing people postpartum are safe for nursing and should be used in whatever amount is recommended by the doctor and that controls your pain. Pain can impact milk transfer, delay birth recovery, and impact bonding. Moreover, I like you, and I don't want you to be in unnecessary pain. Feeding positions can help mitigate pain. If the position you are using makes pain worse, see the positions section (page 107) or call in the feeding team to help you find a way to sit or lie down that minimizes your pain.

MEDICAL CRISIS

Sometimes a baby or birthing person has a full medical crisis during birth. If this happens, feeding takes a back seat, and know that we will revisit these aspects of your baby's care when everyone is stable. Babies can have formula or donor milk while you recover. You can pump while your baby recovers.

So what can you do with this information if you can't control birth? You can give birth in the place that feels safest to you with providers you trust. For some people, that's a home birth, for some it is an operating room, and there is no moral difference between them.

If nursing is extremely important to you and you need a starting place, consider looking for Baby Friendly accredited birth places in your area.

What does "Baby Friendly" mean when it comes to birth place? Baby friendly is a WHO accreditation that birth places can go through to make sure they are knowledgeable and skilled in supporting breastfeeding. The WHO has done years of research on what medical guidelines help families get off to a best possible start and have the best shot at successful nursing if that's their goal. However, be aware that some of them require a waiver to offer formula, just as they would for donor milk, and/or they may be more reluctant to use bottles. Some of the practices can come off as formula-shaming, particularly at a very sensitive point in your life. However, these establishments on the whole have more tools to help with all kinds of infant feeding, and you have my permission to fully tune out any "breast is best" nonsense that comes along with that.

WHAT TO PACK

Here are my recommendations for your hospital bag, but just know that if baby comes before you are packed, the hospital has everything you truly need.

Have a separate postpartum bag from your birth bag. This bag can stay in the car or in a corner until after baby has arrived and it will keep your creature comforts from getting mixed up. Birth books will cover your birth bag pretty well. Here is what goes in your postpartum bag:

If you're planning on nursing:

- Comfortable tops and clothes with easy access to your chest
- Some kind of nipple cream for healing. This can be anything from Vaseline to a special marketed nipple cream. Research shows they all promote healing the same way.
- A nursing pillow (bed pillows work great, but I find that if you have the choice of bringing anything with you, the travel My Brest Friend travel pillow is nice to have)

If you want to formula feed or are undecided about it:

- Most birthing places have formula, but if you want to use one you've selected, then bring some with you, along with a few bottles.

If you are giving birth and plan to exclusively formula feed:

- Some people know from before birthing their baby that they do not want to do any nursing. If that's you, you will want to talk to your medical team about the best way to stop milk production. Your body will go ahead with a milk transition regardless, and that can cause pain or infection if you aren't removing milk. Some medical teams may suggest prescription medications.
- You can also use the lymphatic drainage massages on page 117 and Sudafed. Because decongestants dry up mucus membranes, they can also be helpful in drying up milk production.

If you'll be bottle feeding and are adopting/having a surrogacy birth:

- They will have formula there, but if you'd like to use your own, go ahead and bring it with you, along with a few bottles.
- If you are traveling to the birth of your baby, bring extra bottles, dish soap, and a wash basin with you to wash bottles wherever you are staying until you travel home.

A NOTE ON CIRCUMCISION

Whether or not to circumcise your baby is a personal and cultural choice. Circumcision is commonly done with a topical anesthetic and sugar water on a pacifier for comfort. Sucking and sugar have been shown to be effective pain relief for newborns. That being said, it is stressful for a baby to undergo a small surgery and be separated from parents; this combined with a bit of a sugar crash from the pain-relief glucose tends to result in a very sleepy baby in the six to twelve hours after the procedure. Be sure to do a nice big feeding before the procedure and expect your baby to be sleepy after. If your baby is having trouble eating, you may want to wait a few days and do the circumcision as an outpatient procedure.

Feeling prepared? Only joking. No one does. It's good to think about what you want, but be open to the plan changing. That goes for your birth plan and your feeding plan alike.

CHAPTER 9

THE FOURTH TRIMESTER (THE FIRST THREE MONTHS)

Your baby is here. Hopefully they are in your arms, but maybe they are in a NICU. I think of this time almost like a Christmas tree lighting festival. After much anticipation, preparation, and hard work, the switch is thrown and the world lights up. People gather to *oooh* and *ahhh*. Suddenly, you are a parent or are a parent again.

Getting pregnant and being pregnant may have been straightforward, or maybe it was incredibly difficult. Maybe you've adopted or had a baby via surrogacy. These processes are all laborious, but now the real hard work begins. Babies do not come with instructions, but they are good communicators. Your work in the days, weeks and months to come is to get to know this brand-new person and learn to listen to and respond to them. For newborns, most of that caring and responding will be feeding them.

THE BABY IS HERE, HOURS 0–5

FOR BREAST-FED BABIES: 1–2 feedings in the first 5 hours of life
FOR BOTTLE-FED BABIES: About half an ounce per feeding

The hour after birth, sometimes called "the golden hour" is a very intense time for our bodies and minds. Your baby is looked over, the placenta is delivered, things settle down, and at some point in that hour, your baby eats. Physiologically for your baby, they suddenly go from being completely cared for by someone else's body via the placenta to having to regulate their own temperature, breathe, and eat all on their own. It is a very big adjustment.

Babies can get a little help doing those things through skin-to-skin, a.k.a. a baby's bare skin against another person's bare skin. When babies are skin-to-skin, they regulate temperature, breathing, and even blood sugar better, as they are born to coregulate, which means their breathing and temperature follow yours. When they are near, their stress goes down and they can manage their blood sugar better. It's one of the most incredible things in all of nature.

Sometimes skin-to-skin isn't possible, or not possible with you. If babies need medical assistance during this time, they are warmed and regulated by other tools that work great. If you need medical assistance, or even just need a post-birth moment, partners can do skin-to-skin instead, and if you don't have a partner, a nurse can hold your baby until you're ready. Don't worry—this special magic doesn't expire after an hour. You will get lots of time to hold your baby, help reduce their stress, calm their body, and slow their breathing.

Physiologically, this is also an incredibly intense and transitional time for the birthing person. The uterus now needs to quickly shrink down, pass the placenta and start closing off the open wound it leaves behind. From your providers' perspective, this is the hardest part. One of the ways that we make sure that the uterus starts shrinking back down is by engaging the contraction hormones: oxytocin, or its synthetic counterpart, Pitocin. Medical teams may also "massage" your abdomen to make sure this process goes according to plan. While all this is happening, a baby nursing releases natural oxytocin, which helps the uterus contract. And yes, this juggling act of hormones, medical observation, bonding, feeling, and learning to feed a baby is as messy of a traffic jam as it sounds.

After a cesarean birth, your baby is delivered and either placed on your chest or brought for you to see. Some people feel ready to have some skin-to-skin time, but many don't. Partners who feel up for baby-holding can do skin-to-skin instead. If you don't have a partner, then a nurse will assist. Once a birthing person has been transferred from the operating surface into a bed for transport to a recovery room, they are often more ready to greet their baby. Some people have big feelings about cesarean birth because of a fear that it will irreparably change their nursing experience. This just isn't true. Cesareans are a normal way to birth, and they do not mean you are destined to not meet your feeding goals.

Remember, birth is intense, whether surgical or vaginal. Maybe you needed/used pain-management drugs during your labor. Maybe you haven't eaten in a day or three. Plus, you've been waiting months to meet this person. All of this is to say, it is extremely normal to be very overwhelmed during this time.

Some common descriptions of this time (for birthing and non-birthing parents):

- Overwhelmed
- Nauseous
- Shaking
- Pain
- Joy
- Exhaustion
- Not bonded
- Full of love
- Weak
- Hungry
- Disoriented
- Disassociated
- Relieved

It is okay to feel however you feel and to take care of yourself. Your baby does not need to immediately nurse. Synthetic oxytocin, known as Pitocin, can be used to medically manage uterine contractions and bleeding if necessary. Partners can do skin to skin. Babies can rest happily in warmers. It is okay to need a minute.

You may also feel very excited about and fiercely protective about spending this time with your baby. That's okay, too. There is no right way to feel after birth.

Hold your baby and get to know each other when you are ready and able.

The missing hours

For me, instead of a golden hour, there are missing hours. My memories are a hazy mix of twilight and confusion. Like some of you, my kiddo had to go right to the NICU. Some of you maybe had to do a medical recovery yourself. We are not all "happy and healthy" after birth. We are a valid and important part of the birth continuum. It doesn't serve any of us to block out these possible outcomes. We are often shamed into the corners: no one wants to hear our scary stories. But our stories are real, they are important, they can help others. If you had a traumatic birth, I hope that my story has helped you.

A NOTE ON POST-BIRTH SEPARATION

If you and your baby are separated after birth because your baby needs medical attention, you can hand express or pump to build a milk supply for when your baby is ready.

If you and your baby are separated after birth because you need medical care, you can have someone else do skin to skin and feed them. Prioritize your recovery and work through feeding later. Milk is replaceable; you are not, and you deserve to be well.

These are uncommon but gut-wrenching situations. Know from my experience that your first feeding will be your first feeding, even if it isn't how you pictured it, or is weeks after your baby is born. Our memories of our babies are part of our unique stories, and just because it wasn't movie perfect doesn't make it not right or not good.

BABY'S FIRST HUNGER CUES

Babies are often a little stunned themselves after being born. Most babies will start to acclimate a bit in the first hour or so and warm up to the idea of wanting to eat. You'll get your very first glimpse of "hunger cues." Cues are ways that babies communicate with us, an inborn set of reflexes that comes standard with all babies. Hunger cues are how a baby indicates they are ready to eat. Babies will start to look around, bring their hands to their mouths and start bobbing up and down like little birds pecking around for food. Midwives and labor and delivery nurses are uniquely skilled at facilitating this first feeding. If I'm being honest, sometimes they are a little too good and will smash a latch before you even know what is happening, so there is no need to worry too much about having to manage this very first feeding on your own. And also, some of this time might just be a blur that you ride out. Learn more about hunger cues on page 190 and about latching on page 99.

PARTNERS

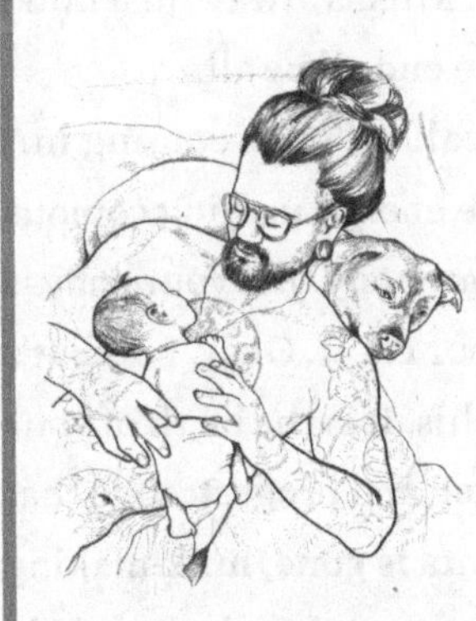

Go ahead and become an expert in observing hunger cues. Watching your baby for these signals can really help your responsiveness and bond. If you are doing a bottle feeding, watch for early cues to go ahead and prep a bottle. If your partner is nursing the next feeding, give them the heads up that it's a good time to go pee, get a snack, and get prepped for a feeding.

If you are planning to exclusively bottle feed

If you are going bottles all the way, you will get a bottle ready when your baby starts to cue. Hospitals provide formula, so you can request it. This will most likely be a bottle of premixed sterile formula. They will have slow-flow nipples you attach right to that bottle and feed. If you feel specific about providing your own formula, I would recommend bringing a container of formula and a bottle of your choosing (refer to page 138). The smallest Dr. Brown's bottle is my preferred option based on size and flow rate. This is only for term babies; preterm babies need to have sterile formula overseen by their doctors.

Newborn babies' tummies are very small at this point, so half an ounce will do. It is tricky to paced bottle feed such small volumes, so let your baby do a bit of sucking before tipping milk into their mouth and then tip the bottle back so that a feeding takes at least ten minutes. More info on paced bottle feeding on page 144.

Milk transition

During pregnancy and right after birth, your body makes milk, but it's extra high in protein and low in water; this is known as *colostrum*. This is just the right fit for the tiny tummies of frequently eating newborns. People sometimes get worried about colostrum because it isn't "real milk," I assure you, it is; it is just very dense. On the other hand, it is also sometimes elevated to being the most important, valuable milk. Milk is always just milk. Renewable, species-specific, and cool, but not the end all be all.

Giving birth signals a process that is often called "milk coming in." While you are pregnant, your body doesn't waste energy making copious amounts of milk, so a hormone "cascade" tells your body that your baby is here, and your body should now feed them via your chest. Okay, I lied: It's not actually the birth of your baby that triggers this. It is the birth of your placenta. The placenta gives off signals for estrogen and progesterone that tell your body to not make milk. Once the placenta is gone, milk-making hormones have a clear path to transition from colostrum (condensed early milk) into a bigger volume of more diluted milk.

If you are nursing or pumping, now is the time to get milk moving. The key to the first few days is: Small volumes very often. This is by design. These small, frequent feedings help your body figure out how much milk to make. If you are a visual learner, check out the graph on page 282.

When your pregnancy hormones go down your milk hormones can spike. Unlike pregnancy hormones, these are not constant; they are triggered by nipple stimulation. That means that for your body to get the signal to transition milk and establish a full production you need to spike these hormones eight to twelve times in twenty-four hours, which is about how often your baby will want to eat. Notice that I did not say every two to three hours. Your baby should wake at various intervals in a day, sometimes you might do fifteen minutes of feeding, or sometimes your baby will take a three-hour break to rest. The important metric is the number of times in twenty-four hours, not the time between them. If your baby is too sleepy to wake up for all eight to twelve feedings and is losing excessive weight, your team may recommend a more rigid feeding schedule. But start out by following cues and tracking feeds per twenty-four hours.

If you are planning to exclusively pump

Colostrum is very difficult to pump because of the small volumes and the honeylike consistency. If you can't nurse or don't want to nurse but still want to get milk production going, you can either hand express into a spoon and give that to your baby or pump as a workout for your hormones and brain and just not worry about volume.

If long-term exclusive pumping is your goal, I recommend five minutes of hand expression and ten minutes of pumping to get those hormone spikes in the graph on page 282.

If you are planning to nurse

Babies are born with certain reflexes to help them smell their way to a chest and latch on. That being said, they are still uncoordinated, and they are rarely very good at it. You can absolutely leave your baby skin to skin, low on your chest, and let them work their way toward nursing, or you can help them along (see latching techniques on page 101). It's also common for a midwife, nurse, or lactation consultant to step in and maneuver your chest into a baby's mouth with great precision but not a lot of communication. Ideally, they will place their hands over yours and talk you through how to latch a baby.

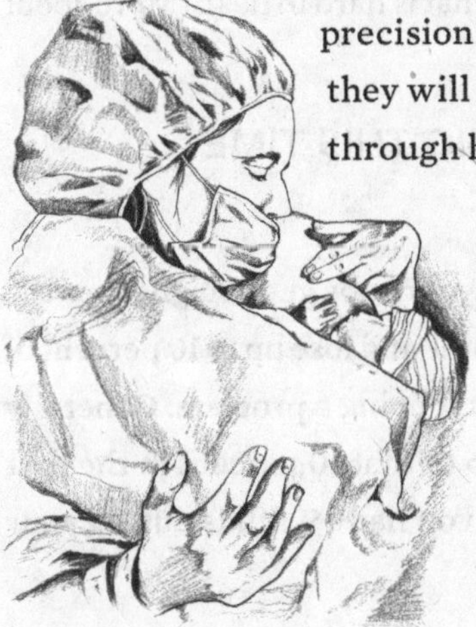

This first feeding can feel very intense. Emotionally and physically. This might be a fully new sensation. Most parents have some worry about whether or not it is "working." Feel free to ask your nurses or midwife for reassurance.

Some things you might feel during this first feeding:

- A sense of chaos, like you don't know what you are doing
- Magical calm
- Dysphoria
- Anxiety
- Nipple tugging
- Nipple pain (remember, while common, this is your body telling you to ask for help)

Signs that milk is moving:

- Dry mouth
- Being overcome with sleepiness
- Painful uterine contractions

How to take a baby off

What should your nipple feel like? It should feel like tugging. It should not feel like pinching, rubbing, or shooting pain. If it does, ask for help. To take a baby off, put your finger in their mouth along the gums to pop the suction. Keeping your finger in their mouth, pull your baby away and then try again for a better latch. (For more on unlatching, see page 103.)

It is important not to nurse through pain, even during this very first feeding. Painful nursing can cause damage that is hard to heal. (More about pain and latching on page 103.)

MORE ABOUT YOUR BABY DURING THIS TIME

The 10 percent guidepost

Sometime in this hour is also usually when your baby gets weighed for the first time. Babies are born with extra fat stores and lose up to 10 percent of their weight in the first two weeks without it being a problem. Generally speaking, we expect a term baby to lose up to that 10 percent in the first week and gain it back the second week. If you had IV fluids during your birth, you may want to ask for another weight a few hours later, once your baby has peed off the excess fluid they received through your IV. This will give you a more accurate picture of how they are doing with feeding based on weight gain or loss.[18]

Blood sugar

One of the things we worry about with newborns is high or low blood sugar. Because of this, babies who have risk factors—late preterm, large for gestational age, small for gestational age, or carried by someone with gestational diabetes—may need to have their blood sugar checked at birth. Unfortunately, this is often done without a first feeding and away from parents, which doesn't give your baby their best chance at maintaining a healthy blood sugar level. This can trigger a complex set of interventions that is sometimes necessary, but can sometimes be avoided by doing a heel prick during skin-to-skin. It's worth asking your doctor if they will do this. Ask that the blood sugar check be taken while baby is skin-to-skin (ideally with the birthing person) and after a feeding. If you want to be extra sure that your baby has a good chance of stabilizing their blood sugar, you can hand express milk (colostrum) into a spoon and tip it into their mouth a few minutes before the blood test.

Preterm babies

Whether your baby was born early for their reasons or yours, it is very overwhelming to have such a small baby. Preemies go immediately to a NICU or special-care nursery to be looked after. It can feel lonely to be without your baby during this time. You will be asked to pump milk by your medical team soon after birth; this allows you to build a milk supply regardless of if your baby is ready to eat or not. Depending on your baby's (or babies') medical status and age, they may start with just IV nutrition or begin receiving food via a tube in their nose. This allows babies to take in nutrition to grow without using calories to eat, but they will work on that skill when they are ready.

PREEMIE DIGESTION

Scientifically, this is the one instance where the health outcomes for formula- and breast-milk-fed babies are crystal clear: exclusive formula is less safe for preterm babies. Preterm babies do not have fully formed and lined guts, because they are not yet designed for digestion. This leaves them prone to gut infections that are very dangerous. The best prevention we have found is breast milk. Many parents find the demands of getting to a NICU, taking care of other aspects of their life, and pumping very difficult to manage. Do what you can while doing your best to manage your mental health and life. For others, it feels like the one thing you can actually DO to participate in your baby's medical care. Follow what works for you, knowing that if you aren't able to produce enough milk for your baby, you can ask the NICU for donor milk (see page 74 for more on donor milk). Milk banks collect, test, and pasteurize milk from other parents who have extra for this very purpose.

Preterm milk as it is expressed from a parent's body is different from mature milk. It has a higher amount of protein and a lower amount of lactose. Babies produce more lactase (the enzyme that breaks down lactose) as they reach forty weeks' gestation. Our bodies know to makes milk that is easier for preemies to digest. Formula makers follow this lead and make specialized formulas for preemies that are lower in lactose and higher in overall calories to make sure these babies get what they need. This is a good option if parental or donor milk isn't available for your preemie or in medical circumstances where it is recommended. If you aren't producing milk, your neonatologist may recommend switching to a preemie formula from human milk after a certain age or after reaching other markers of health and maturity.

Babies tend to get their food via feeding tube until at least 32 weeks, so before this time they are fed expressed milk or formula, and a product called a "fortifier" is added to it.

Preemies also need more iron than term babies. Your neonatologist and pediatrician will keep a close eye on your baby's iron levels and may recommend vitamin drops with iron.

As preemies approach forty weeks, they will work on eating by mouth (instead of a nasogastric tube) and growing. During this time the fortifiers and other supplements will be phased out based on your baby's health and as they develop digestion similar to that of a term baby.

Discharge from the NICU

And so begins a whole new adventure. From here on out, you take an active role in feeding and caring for your baby, instead of your body or a NICU team making sure your baby gets what they need. Your baby is ready to be in your care, and you have everything you need to care for them. The underlying principle of this book is "enoughness." You are enough whether you make enough milk or don't. Formula and human milk are both food. As you move on from pregnancy into this transition, listen to your baby. Listen to your gut. You are enough whether you are bringing home one baby or three. You are enough if you had the birth of your dreams or a birth you would never have chosen. You are enough if you pump, if you bottle feed, if you are still recovering, if you need support for your mental health. And now, let's learn how to do all of these things.

THE FIRST SEVEN DAYS

FOR BREAST-FED BABIES: **8–12 feeds over 24 hours**
FOR BOTTTLE-FED BABIES: **From around approx. 5–7 mL increasing to 60–81 mL per feeding; or from approx. 1 to 3 ounces per feeding**

From birth until around day seven, your baby gradually increases the volume they eat. As milk transitions, it goes from being sticky and low in volume to thin and more of what people visualize as milk. If you want to provide milk for your baby but don't want to/can't nurse, hand expression works better than pumping at this stage (see previous chapter on how to do it).

If you gave birth, you will still be recovering. Expecting someone to do such a major recovery while caring for a new life is ridiculous, and I'm so sorry. Get as much support as you can so you can get as much rest as you can. Stay on top of your pain management and don't try to tough it out or do everything yourself. You may also experience engorgement if you are nursing, which can be painful. See page 117 for how to relieve this.

Some important things to prioritize in this first week are:

- Is your baby eating enough?
- Are you eating enough?
- Do you have comfortable places to feed your baby and sleep?
- Is your pain being well managed?
- If you are nursing, is nursing painful? Do you need more help?
- How is your mood?

BABY BLUES

The baby blues are a way that people refer to the normal drop many experience when their hormones change after birth. This usually happens between three and twelve days after birth or a miscarriage and makes people feel weepy and have mood swings. Baby blues are well remedied with some good sleep and fresh air. If your mood doesn't bounce back easily, you can't sleep, or you are very anxious, something more serious is going on. Please check in with yourself now and often, and see page 253 for more on mood.

BABY WEIGHT

Term babies are born with healthy fat stores to get them through the early days of figuring out how to eat. Babies are weighed soon after birth, and then we give them about a 10 percent weight loss buffer for the next two weeks. That is to say, we expect newborns to lose weight. The Academy of Breastfeeding Medicine says that we should wait until that 10 percent mark and consider all the factors before we intervene. If you are nursing, giving your baby milk you didn't make in the first few weeks of life can throw off the supply-and-demand chain of feeding. So, rest assured that there is no medical indication to supplement until your baby has lost a full 10 percent, and even then consider: Is your baby otherwise healthy? Are your feedings improving? Is your milk transitioning? Is your baby eating eight to twelve times per day? If so, stay the course, weight should start trending up in the next twenty-four hours. There is no nee to keep track unless your care provider tells you to do so. I d one extra weight check for nursing families when baby is six This is an important moment in milk transition and can catch w issues that often appear between the one- and two-month ped rician visits. Just ask your provider to schedule a nurse visit for a weight check on week six of life for extra peace of mind.

BABY SLEEPING AND EATING CYCLES

Newborns mostly live in a perpetual cycle of eating and sleeping. These cycles will eventually stretch out and consolidate into more predictable naps and feedings. In the early days, though, you just have to go along for the ride. Following your baby's cues is the best way to learn what your baby needs and help them eat the right amount for their body. For nursing parents, it also helps you make the right amount of milk for your baby.

Learning to read cues

As nonspeaking creatures, babies mostly communicate through their body language or as we call them, *cues*. Cues are ways that your baby tells you they are ready to eat, sleep, even poop if you care to pay close enough attention. These cues are a combination of reflexes and instincts that communicate a need. This is why the World Health Organization (WHO) has begun recommending "rooming in" with your baby. This means that our baby stays close to you instead of in another room with nurses and other babies while in the hospital. In their research the WHO found that when babies stayed with their parents, they gained weight faster because parents learned how to know when they were hungry and feed them more quickly. Babies also cried less, and parents felt more confident that they could care for their babies when they went home. This time together gives parents a chance to learn these cues as quickly as possible. The theory here is that if you are only ever brought a very hungry baby, you never learn what precedes that moment. Rooming-in helps build responsive relationships. Will there still be times when you have no earthly clue what is going on? Absolutely. Nevertheless, listening to your baby's body language will help you anticipate needs and get off on the right foot.

Hunger cues

Babies under the age of six weeks cycle continuously from sleeping to eating and back to sleeping again. Babies begin their waking cycle by giving early hunger cues.

1. **Eye flutters:** As they come up into light sleep, their eyelids will flutter, and you will see their eyes begin to move under their closed eyelids.
2. **Searching:** Next, babies will start to look around, opening their eyes and turn from side to side.
3. **Rooting:** Your baby begins to try to eat anything nearby, bobbing up and down or bringing their hands to their mouth. Soon, with eyes open wide, the rooting begins to get more frantic, like a chicken pecking for seeds. This is an ideal time to get going on the feeding. If you aren't ready to go, you had best hurry.
4. **Crying:** This is what we call a late feeding cue. Eating is a new and complicated skill for newborns, and they can get very frustrated if they are trying to eat at this point of hunger. They will sometimes scream and seem to refuse food. This just means they are too hungry to get themselves settled to eat. If possible, try snuggling, bouncing, and shushing to calm your baby down before starting the feeding, as frantic crying feeds can lead to swallowing air and frustration for everyone. You can also give a clean finger to suck on to calm them down and get them organized.

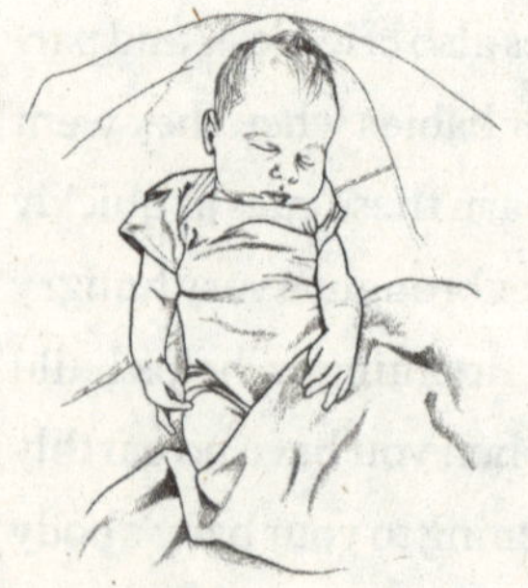

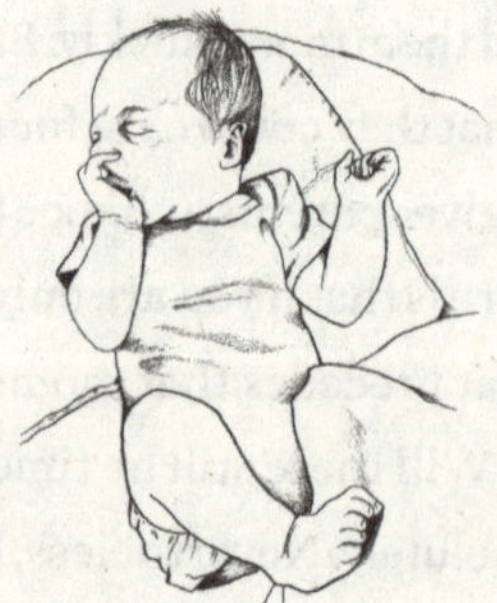

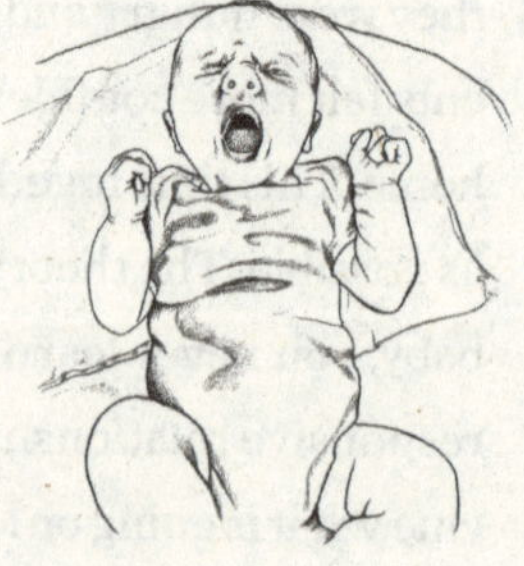

CREATING YOUR FEEDING ZONES

It is really important to make a zone or two that are comfortable to feed in. This might be a rocker you carefully picked out; it might also just be your bed.

You need a seating surface you can easily get into and out of and enough blankets and pillows. Basically, a set up that takes pressure off any injured areas in your crotch or midsection.

Feeding floppy little newborns takes some setup, so noticing these earlier cues gives you a chance to fix a bottle if you're bottle feeding, and to set up pillows and grab a snack and water before things get too desperate.

Something like 400 percent of toddler and parent meltdowns are due to low blood sugar. Beginning to understand your child's early hunger and fullness cues is a good skill to apply to yourself and your kiddo as they grow.

Sucks, swallows and eating cues

Your baby also gives you important signals while they eat. You can watch closely and listen for swallows. If they are swallowing after every suck, they are eating very quickly. If they aren't doing many swallows at all, they might be sleeping.

Notice how when your baby is eating, their jaw moves slightly up and down a few times followed by a "kah" sound and a big drop of the jaw. That is a swallow. This pattern of suck, swallow, breathe is complex but innate to most babies. Others need some help getting the hang of it.

Babies come hard wired with three different suck patterns:

Fast, fast, fast sucks at the beginning of a feeding. These firm, fast sucks are designed to get in a good organized rhythm before milk starts flowing, and in nursing parents, triggers the nerves in the nipple and breast to start making milk.

Suck, suck, swallow, breathe. These big steady sucks, or as I sometimes call them, "piston sucks," are like a mechanical pump. There are a few big draws before dropping the jaw down and swallowing. This is where the majority of actual eating happens. Observing these swallows has been shown to be an effective way to calculate milk transfer. So, if you're nursing, watching for these can be reassuring that your baby is actively eating.

Suck, flutter, suck, flutter. These little sucks remind me of a butterfly flapping its wings. These passive, "non-nutritive" sucks are a sign that your baby is no longer eating and has moved on to soothing. This is your cue to check in and see if your baby seems to have eaten enough (fullness cues, below) or if you need to wake them up to go back to the big sucks and finish the feeding.

The butterfly sucks can get us into trouble when we are feeding based on the clock instead of paying attention to how a baby is eating. Imagine yourself on a warm beach with your book. You start to slightly doze off. Your arms loosen and you almost drop your book, realizing you are falling asleep you jerk awake to read a few more pages, only to doze off again a few pages later. This is sort of how newborns feed, and the younger or more preterm the baby, the sleepier. You are a beach to them. Nice and cozy, baby will start to relax into a feeding and doze off. If they do this before they are actually done eating, try undressing baby to their diaper and use baby sit-ups and shoulder presses to wake them back up.

WHEN IS THE FEEDING OVER?

Many parents come into my office frazzled and desperate, accompanied by a novel's worth of notes on feedings. They have set up to feed their baby only to realize they don't have their phone handy to hit "go" on their trusted feeding app. I love each of them for their dutiful commitment to data. I'm married to a data scientist. I love data. The problem is that when it comes to feeding babies, qualitative data is much more useful than quantitative data. (There is a feeding tracker on page 281 to help you keep qualitative data on feedings.)

With bottle-fed babies, it is easy to know they are gaining enough. Your medical team gives you a volume based on weight, and you go up or down from there based on if your baby seems hungry more often or spits up large volumes after feeds.

With nursing babies, it can be much harder and akin to cooking in a pressure cooker. With no way to peek in and stir the pot, it can be nerve-racking. So, pees, poops, and weight checks are the only ways to know your baby is eating well.

TRACKING FEEDINGS VS. UNDERSTANDING THEM

I do not recommend timing feedings. Instead, track number of feedings per twenty-four hours. A clock cannot tell you if your baby has eaten, and you need to look at your baby and body to know if you did a full feeding. A clock cannot tell you if your baby has eaten a full feeding. For that information you need to look at your baby. Babies can absolutely butterfly suck for twenty minutes, taking in very little milk, or can guzzle a full feeding in four minutes. I cannot overstate how useless amount of time is in figuring out intake. The point of tracking feedings is making sure that your baby is eating eight to twelve times per day. That is all the quantitative data you need. You can track with tallies on a piece of paper, or a notes app (if you would rather have it on your phone), or use my feeding tracker on page 281.

The duration of a feeding Does. Not. Matter. Many parents are told that to nurse a baby, you feed them for fifteen to twenty minutes on one side, then fifteen to twenty minutes on the other. Then repeat every three hours. This is FALSE. I don't know who started this, or who makes the breastfeeding apps, but timing feedings is not a good way to tell how feedings are going. In fact, following cue-based feedings is so superior to timed ones that it made it into the WHO Ten Steps to Effective Breastfeeding that underpin Baby Friendly Accreditataon. When we respond to hunger cues, a few very important things happen:

- We develop secure attachment by responding to our babies.
- Our babies learn the feeling of their own hunger and satiety which is foundational to our lifelong relationship to food.
- We see less engorgement, less mastitis, and better weight gain.

- We don't waste time and energy trying to force a feeding on a baby who isn't ready to eat yet.

The number that is important to know is how many times a baby woke up to eat in the last twenty-four hours. If a baby is not waking up to eat eight to twelve times in twenty-four hours, something could be wrong and your pediatrician needs to know.

THINGS TO NOTICE AT THIS STAGE

Fullness cues

Hungry babies are tight little balls of tension. Hands in the mouth, tight clenched fists. As a baby eats, their body will relax into a pose like a T. rex holding arms up halfway. Halfway through a feeding, many babies will doze off having had a snack, enough to comfortably snooze for twenty minutes only to wake again acting like they are starving. A very full baby has fully open, relaxed hands and arms. You should be able to pick up an arm and let it drop right to their side with no resistance, like a wet noodle. You can also brush your knuckle along the face of a fully fed baby and get no response, whereas a hungry baby will try to root for just about any stimulus.

You can also watch your baby for swallows. This has been shown to be a very good indicator of how much milk a baby is eating. Swallows sounds like a soft "kah" sound, and you can see your baby's tongue muscle drop when it happens by watching for a bullfrog-like drop under their chin (see page 191 for QR code).

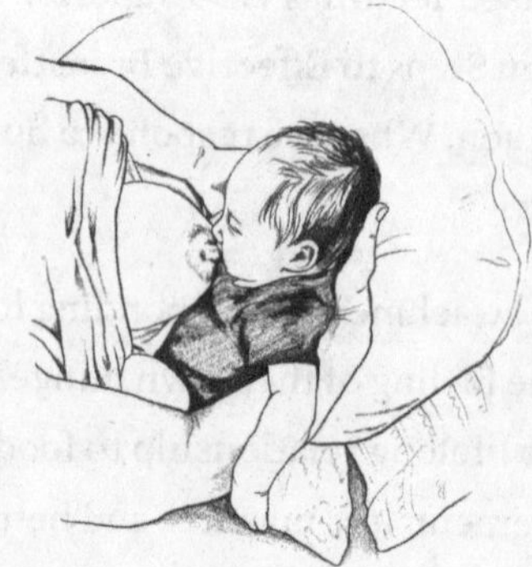

Learning when your breasts are full and drained

When you begin a nursing session, touch your chest. Just notice it. This must be what full feels like for you. This interoception (sense of your own body) will develop over time, but it is a valuable skill to learn. This is your best way to know if your baby or pump drained your milk well. Don't expect to know what to feel for right away, but over time, you will feel it.

This sensation gets more subtle around the six-week mark, but for now you will feel a change from firm feeling to soft feeling.

DRAIN ONE SIDE, THEN OFFER THE NEXT.

While you are feeding your baby, observe them. You are looking for qualitative data, remember? Now, think back to those three kinds of sucks. You are looking for those big, productive bullfrog sucks. Check if your baby slips into butterfly sucks. Feel your chest: Still firm? Wake them up by pressing them into you with your palm at the shoulder; this should remind them to keep sucking vigorously. You can also use the back of your hand to "scrape the brownie batter" and slide milk toward them (page 162). These two techniques usually jumpstart a baby back into action; if not, fishhook (page 103) to pop them off, and then wake them up with baby sit-ups or a diaper change and relatch when awake.

But wait! The same side or is it time to switch? Feel your breasts. If the side baby was nursing on still feels firm all around or in some areas, then

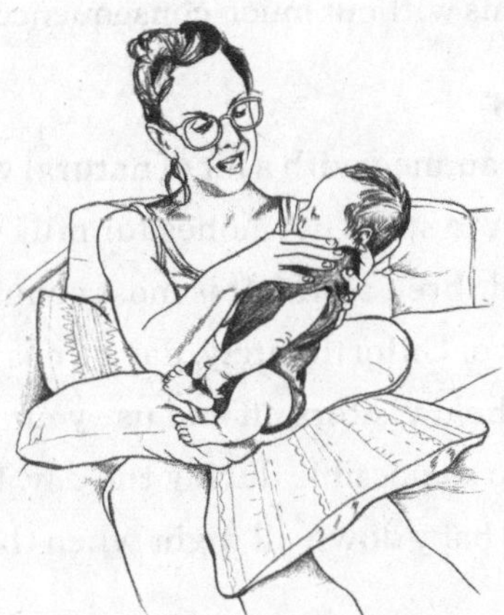

go right back to that breast. If it feels nice and soft all around, but baby still seems hungry (see hunger cues, page 190), switch sides.

Some people do a full feeding on one side, or even two feedings on one side before moving to the next. Some people do three sides per feeding (right, left, back to the right), thus catching the milk produced by the energy building up while they were nursing on the other side. At times (usually in the evening) babies will go back and forth and back and forth, catching the little bits of milk produced by a charge up in your breast while they were on the other side. This back and forth is called "cluster feeding" and is your baby filling up for a longish chunk of sleep. Ideally, you would put on a good season of TV and nurse, nurse, nurse, expecting to go to sleep once they are done, so you can catch every moment that cluster earned you. If your baby seems to cluster feed like this around the clock you should check in with a lactation professional.

Clusters aside, healthy term babies eat every one to five hours, with different spacing at different times of the day. What matters is that they are eating enough times per day, not how these feedings are spaced. If your baby was planning on a four-hour break and you try to wake her up at the three-hour mark, that will be a very frustrating and sleepy feeding. If your baby decided it was time to eat at the two-hour mark and you wanted to stretch it to three, you will have a very hangry baby on your hands. The goal is to learn their cues and learn your body for the first six weeks while your production settles. After that, you can nudge toward a schedule and add in pumping sessions without much consequence to your production.

The day 2/3 cluster

Babies come preprogrammed with a lot of natural wisdom. One of these wisdom is the instinct to spike hormones for milk transition sometime between days two and three of life. It is most common for this to occur on the night of day two. Unfortunately, day two is also when everyone wants to visit. Try to hold visitors off and use your Do Not Disturb sign to catch as much sleep as possible during the day. It is very common to not be able to set your baby down all night when they are doing this big cluster feeding.

Pees and poops

Another way to check if your baby is eating enough is through the contents of their diaper. When babies are first born, their stomachs are very small. This is a perfect match for the small amounts of milk that are produced in the early days. As a birthing person goes through a hormone transition over the first week after a baby is born, they gradually make a larger milk volume that is more watered down. This early milk is very diuretic and has tons of immune factors to line the gut. One of the jobs of this early milk is to get the gut moving and push out the meconium. Meconium is tar like early poop that is made up of broken-down amniotic fluid and red blood cells. Over the first week of life, the poop of human milk–fed babies turns bright yellow. Formula is digested differently than breast milk. If you are exclusively formula feeding, you will see a switch from black, thick tar to a looser light-brown poop.

The color and number of poops is how we track feedings in breast-fed babies, for whom we cannot see how much is going in; so instead we watch how much is coming out.

It is helpful, though gross, to see this in color. You can see a poop color chart on page 282 or use the following QR code:

JAUNDICE

I know, we are talking about poop—why am I bringing up jaundice? Jaundice is extremely common in newborns: about two thirds of babies have it at some point. You may notice your baby becoming jaundiced if their skin begins to yellow, or they aren't pooping enough. A good place to look for yellowness is the sclera, or whites of your baby's eyes, which are a bit more foolproof than the range of skin colors. When our bodies break down red blood cells, they are broken apart, and one of these parts is called *bilirubin*. This bilirubin then goes into our intestines and comes out in poop. Newborns have an unusual little enzyme called UGT1A1, which lets the gut take the bilirubin back up into the bloodstream. This is completely normal and is known as *physiological jaundice*, and happens a few weeks after birth in babies who eat human milk.

(continues)

Jaundice is checked for with a blood test by your pediatrician.

The second most common kind of jaundice is called *lack-of-breastfeeding jaundice* but you can think of it as "lack-of-pooping" jaundice. This kind of jaundice happens earlier, in the first few days of life, and is a sign that a baby might not be eating enough to stimulate enough pooping. This can cause a frustrating feedback loop where the buildup of bilirubin makes a baby sleepy, which makes them less vigorous eaters, which makes them hard to feed, which causes them to get more jaundiced. At its most extreme, jaundice can be very dangerous, so medical teams treat it rigorously and early.

Signs of jaundice to look for:

- Baby isn't waking for 8–12 feedings per 24 hours
- Baby isn't pooping
- Yellow skin, or yellowing of the whites of the eyes

Treating jaundice

Jaundice is treated with a combination of light therapy and supplementation. The bilirubin buildup will start to show up in a baby's skin, causing some babies to appear yellow. In one of those "woah, science" moments, we can address that bilirubin with a blanket or tanning bed of blue light. Blue light is the highest-energy light, and the photons in blue light are fast enough to destabilize the bilirubin and break it down to address the buildup in the body. Meanwhile, babies with jaundice are given extra food with a syringe or bottle to help make sure they poop out any bilirubin that is in their gut before it has a chance to be taken back up into the bloodstream and circulated. This kind of jaundice is usually treated in a day or two, but it can feel very scary to parents to have their baby taken away and kept in a blue-light incubator. Rest assured that it is very normal and should resolve quickly, but it's a good idea to check in with a lactation professional to protect your production and make a plan to get back to fully nursing after treatment if that's your goal.

Baby pee

Well hydrated babies pee often. The indicator strips on diapers now make it very easy to tell if a baby has peed. Baby pee should be nice and clear. If it starts to look like apple juice, you should check in with your doctor, because that can be an early dehydration sign.

BRICK DUST

This phenomenon of red pee in newborns is caused by an excess of urate crystals and is totally normal and not commonly a sign of dehydration in the first few days, but you should tell your pediatrician anyway just in case. After week one, however, you should contact your doctor about any red or pink showing up in a baby's diapers.

Dehydration

If you have any concern that your baby isn't eating enough, you should have them weighed that day. It is rare for babies to become dehydrated, but it happens, and knowing what to look for can save your baby's life. Whether due to illness, low milk production, or a physiological issue, like pyloric stenosis, dehydration happens, and you should know the signs. If your baby is showing any of these signs, you should go immediately to see a doctor or to an emergency room:

- Dry mouth or eyes
- Depressed fontanel (soft spot on the head)
- Skin tenting (skin stays up in a peak when pinched)
- Dry diaper
- Not waking for feedings

NEWBORN ADVICE FOR NON-BIRTHING AND/OR NON-NURSING PARTNERS

Prepare and present food

I have seen some beautiful plates of one-handed foods in my day. Side tables covered in unwrapped cheese sticks, water bottles and de-stemmed grapes. If you are going to be out of the house for the day, premake a lunch plate and put it on the counter or in the fridge. This ensures that your partner eats a good meal and can do so with one hand. Sometimes, just the barrier of deciding what to eat and serving it keeps us from meeting our needs when we are taking care of little ones.

Get really good at soothing

Babies do a lot of soothing while nursing. You can help your baby expand their soothing tool kit, bond with them, and give your partner a break all at the same time. By building more skills to soothe than nursing, you are preparing your baby for more independent sleep and the ability to be happily looked after by other caregivers. When your baby is done nursing, you can take your baby and practice babywearing, soothing (page 211), or go for a walk around the block together.

Lactation architect

Be observant about your partner's nursing set up. Can you set up the pillows that are needed before your co-parent sits down? Can you spot areas of tension where your partner is holding your baby, but a rolled-up towel could do the job?

Prep bottles/wash pump parts

Pumping is no joke. It takes a lot of time and a lot of energy. Help pitch in with making bottles by really understanding bottle prep and storage and making it your job.

Take care of your mental health

Due to the focus on the birthing person's mental health, it is not uncommon to forget partners. If you don't feel like yourself or need some space to process birth or postpartum, reach out for help. These things are normal, common, and treatable.

WEEKS ONE TO TWO

FOR BREAST-FED BABIES: 8–12 feeds per 24 hours
FOR BOTTLE-FED BABIES: 8–12 bottles (1–3 oz) per 24 hours

Term babies are likely to regain to their birth weight and start steadily gaining through this two-week period. While up to 10 percent weight loss is considered normal in the first two weeks, we look for all of it to be gained back by day fourteen. If not, it's time to intervene. As mentioned before, it's not about how long your baby is feeding or the time between feeds, but whether they are feeding until they are full. See page 191 for sucking patterns and how to know when your baby is full.

Some parents feel ready at this point to start venturing out and about; some people aren't. That's your call. If you are up for it, try going to the home of a friend with a baby or a low-pressure relative: whatever makes you feel most secure.

Two weeks is a good time to take a step back and assess. I know this is a big ask for such a sleep-deprived and stressful time. If you can, talk through what you feel is working and what isn't with a trusted friend or partner.

For formula feeding: How is my baby doing? Is the formula we started with sitting well with them?

For nursing: How is nursing going? Has any pain been resolved? Do we have a solid plan to move forward in a way that works for the whole family? Are there nursing problems that are consistent or that seem to come and go?

For all babies: What is happening with your baby's (or babies') anatomy? Do you notice that they prefer to keep their head to one side or look one way? Do they have a flat spot on their skull? Do they have a heart-shaped tongue or sleep with their mouth open?

Some people who planned to breastfeed may find themselves introducing bottles before this point because it is medically necessary for them or their baby (see necessary supplementation and triple feeding on page 120), but at two weeks I consider nursing "well established" and encourage nursing parents to learn to express milk and start offering bottles and pacifiers.

BUT WHAT ABOUT NIPPLE CONFUSION!?

Nipple confusion is the idea that a baby will like a bottle nipple more than nursing and stop nursing. This is very rare, though some babies develop a flow preference for bottles if we give them too quickly. In my decade of practice and my mentor Ellen Chetwyn's thirty years of practice, we have found that a paced bottle is an excellent tool for teaching, and if you choose a pacifier or bottle nipple that encourages correct sucking position, it can actually strengthen a suck and make it better. Can babies get hooked on bottles and refuse nursing? Absolutely, but it is usually because they are being given the wrong nipple and are drinking too quickly. We also know that pacifiers are good for babies' nervous systems, but they can hide feeding cues in early days, delaying weight gain. Once your baby is back to birth weight or reliably waking up on their own for at least eight feedings a day, a pacifier is a great tool.

HOW TO INTRODUCE BOTTLES TO NURSING BABIES

The goal of this next step is to use your baby's open developmental window to help them learn to eat from a bottle so that you have more flexibility in your life and routines. Not everyone introduces a bottle. If your baby will be reliably with you for the next six months or so and you don't have any desire to bottle feed, that is just fine. Skip this section.

The best way to make sure your baby will take a bottle is to catch them in an open developmental window. Offer a bottle beginning at two to four weeks and then give a bottle at least twice per week thereafter. Keeping your baby used to taking a bottle even when you don't need to ensures that you will have that tool available when you need it. Most families I've worked with find it simplest to find a point in their day when giving a bottle works for their schedule and non-nursing parents seem to enjoy this time for bonding. Some examples of this are: a co-parent gives a bottle to reconnect when they get home from work; a grandparent gives a bottle during the nursing parent's afternoon nap; caregivers split feedings in the night, so the nursing parent gets a longer stretch of sleep while someone else gives a late-night bottle (between 10:00 p.m. and 1:00 a.m.) or an early morning bottle (between 5:00 and 8:00 a.m.).

If you offer a bottle before six weeks and your baby refuses it, it is worth consulting a feeding professional, like a lactation consultant or speech-language pathologist, who, for infants, are the experts in sucking and swallowing. This is unusual, and it would be good to rule out a tie, dysfunctional suck, or cleft. Incorporating bottles can feel like a chaotic addition to a system you just got going, but it is worth it in the long run. After eight to twelve weeks, babies tend to get a little less malleable about feeding, and it can lead to a lot of stress while trying to convince them that taking a bottle so you can take a shower is a good idea. Between two and six weeks, they are just persuadable enough that offering a paced bottle at least two times per week will make it easier to do bottles more often as needed later on.

What bottle/pacifier should I use?

There is an entire market of bottle sample sets and bottles that look/feel/smell like a breast. A bottle is a bottle, not a breast. So, I suggest a narrow-necked bottle that is an appropriate size for your baby's age and has a slow-flow nipple. The nipple should also be long and round. A smashed or bulged shaped nipple will teach your baby to hold their mouth this way which doesn't support their pallet development or sucking skills at this age. These other shaped pacifiers are better left for when your baby is older.

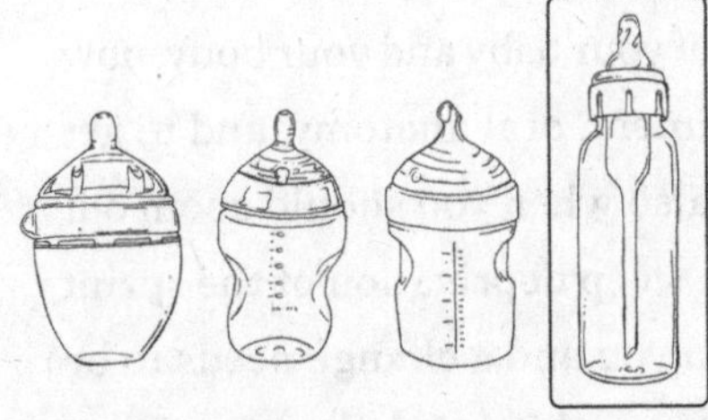

There's much more on choosing a bottle on page 138.

There has been some research that in bottle-fed babies, the bigger the bottle, the more we feed babies. It is human nature to assume a less-full bottle is not enough, so we tend to fill bottles up more and then encourage babies to finish that bottle. This can lead to overfeeding and increased anxiety about pumping enough and bottle preference. We will be starting your young baby on one to three ounces of milk, so a four-ounce bottle is plenty. Once a baby sleeps through the night, they consoli-

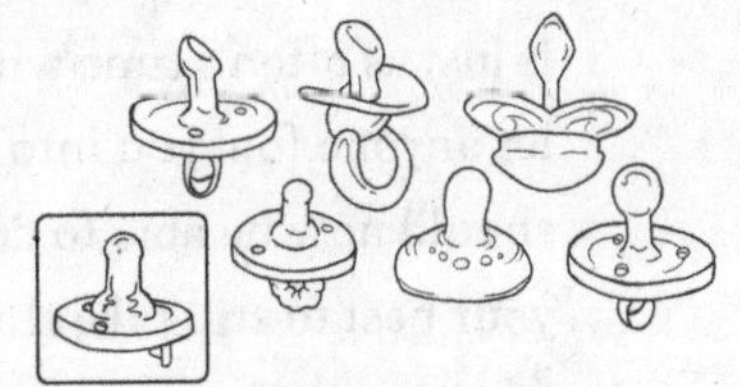

date more of their eating during the day and may need larger bottles. This usually occurs around five to six months at the very earliest.

If nursing is going well and you are planning to both nurse and offer bottles of expressed milk, the two-week mark is a good time to add this in. (Refer to "How to Pump" on page 154 for advice on pumps and pumping.) Usually by this point, you will have found a routine, both of you have learned a good latch, and you are well versed in your baby's cues.

You did it! You made it through the first two weeks as a parent. For many, this is the hardest part until middle school. You juggled huge body changes, your baby's needs, and your own. You probably didn't do it very gracefully. Everyone probably cried a lot. This messiness is also the beauty. I hope you leaned into learning a lot about your baby and finding out what it means to be their parent. Great work, I'm proud of you. Even if things didn't go as planned, and you switched feeding methods entirely and you haven't showered in three days: I am proud of you.

WEEKS THREE TO SIX

FOR BREAST-FED BABIES: 8–12 feedings per 24 hours, still unpredictable in timing

FOR BOTTLE-FED BABIES: 6–12 (2–4 oz) bottles per 24 hours

As you settle into a better understanding of your baby and your body, now is a good time to assess your baby's alignment, oral anatomy, and to get help in those areas if you need it. This is also when you should zoom out and look at the bigger picture. Maybe the sleep deprivation of the sprint through the first few weeks is wearing on you and a change needs to be made. About now, some people feel like they are hitting their stride, but it is just as often a time when people feel like they are hitting a wall. Do not let anyone fool you into thinking your early postpartum is over and you should now be able to do it all. You are still recovering and learning. Do your best to still take things slow. Take naps, stay in pajamas all day, ask friends to come to you.

For you: If you are nursing, this is a good time to take stock of how you are coping both physically and emotionally. Are you feeling any pain? Refer to the "Troubleshooting" section starting on page 115 for common nursing issues.

Regardless of how you are feeding, how is your mood? Let's take stock and dip into the postpartum mood section of this book for check-ins with yourself, as well as with co-parents. As help and attention start to fade and hormones continue to shift, this is a real perinatal mood speed trap. Sleep and mental health are best friends, so it is natural for sleep deprivation to cause depression and anxiety. Are you able to fall asleep when given the opportunity? Do you worry a lot about relatively small things or about big things that are out of your control? Might be time for a mood check.

For your baby: if you haven't already, start tummy time. If you are noticing any oral ties or positional asymmetries (see "Your Baby's Body," beginning on page 46) you should get them looked at.

THE LITTLE-KNOWN SIX-WEEK BREAST TRANSITION

Many people notice that at six weeks postpartum their breasts feel much less intensely full between feedings. They still feel a firmness when it is time to nurse, but it is much less pronounced. In the first six weeks postpartum, your hypothalymus runs the show and sets the tone for your overall milk production by sending hormones from part of your hypothalamus called the *pituitary gland*. This is why your body is so reactive to changes in demand for milk in the first six weeks.

At around six weeks it is almost as though your hypothalamus calls your breasts and says, "I've trained you well. Take it from here." At that point your production is mostly controlled by cues—like FIL (feedback inhibitor of lactation), a protein that signals that you are full and should not make more milk—generated based on how often you drain your breasts.

It's common for people to feel like their production must have evaporated; this isn't the case, it's just your body getting used to the work of making milk. At this point, you will still feel a change in the way your chest feels before and after nursing, but your baby's fullness cues will also help you have a reliable indicator of how they are eating.

At six weeks, when your baby's suck starts to control production instead of your brain, a dysfunctional suck can cause a drop in production. If you are concerned that this is happening, get a weight check from your pediatrician, as well as a pre- and post-feeding weight from a feeding specialist or IBCLC.

REFLUX

Reflux is heartburn. It is extremely common because babies have very weak sphincters (closures) between their stomach and their mouth. The stomach acid from milk coming back up can damage the esophagus, which is very painful. You may be very aware of the need for these sphincters if you have had heartburn in pregnancy. In pregnancy, the hormone relaxin, lack of space, and weaker abdominal muscles let your stomach acid flow upward, and you can feel like a fire-breathing mess when you try to lie down to sleep.

Babies with reflux tend to eat small amounts often and arch as though they are trying to move away from their own throat. There's more on reflux, its causes, and treatment below, but in this instance, you should talk to your baby's doctor.

What we call "reflux" or "spitting up" spans a big spectrum, from a laundry problem to a health problem.

Babies also have little abdominal strength when they are born. Around six months, when your baby can sit up, they will develop the core strength and tone to help keep food where it ought to be.

There are some theories that this baby leakiness is by design, as the sugar and bacteria in fresh human milk can populate the sinuses and help build a baby's immune system. Our knowledge of the microbiome is still far from proving this theory, but I enjoy it even as folklore, because it gives you some reassurance that milk is not wasted when it comes out your baby's nose.

A small amount of spit-up is normal. Spit up will range from thin milk right after eating to chunky milk that has been partially digested later. Spit-up also tends to look like more than it is.

Normal spit-up

- Spits up after some meals but not all.
- Is a small volume, and your baby is gaining weight well.
- Your baby does not seem to be in pain with spitting up.

Spit-up can cross into a medical problem, a.k.a. gastroesophageal reflux disease (GERD) if your baby:

- has a hoarse voice.
- is clearly in pain with spitting up.
- cannot be laid flat without spitting up and seems to be in pain when lying down.
- tends to arch their body excessively or sleep in a backward C-shape, almost as though they are trying to get away from their throat.
- isn't gaining weight well.

If your baby is showing any of these signs, it merits a conversation with your pediatrician. Talk about the risks and benefits of medication, but remember that reflux can cause real (though reversible) damage to the esophagus. The longer it goes untreated, the longer it may take to heal. Reflux medication may also take several weeks to show improvement, due to the damage to the esophagus.

PYLORIC STENOSIS

In our series of valves, the one in the stomach that leads to the intestines is called the *pylorus*. A design flaw where the muscles of this sphincter over-develop. This causes the door to close off, making it impossible to digest milk. This relatively rare condition, called *pyloric stenosis*, masquerades as reflux but is not. If you suspect pyloric stenosis, see your pediatrician or urgent care that day. Symptoms to look out for are:

- Large volumes of regurgitated milk, a whole feeding's worth of milk
- Projectile vomiting
- Lots and lots of crying
- Signs of dehydration: dry eyes, depressed fontanel (soft spot on the head), skin tenting (baby's skin stays up in a peak when pinched)

MAYA'S STORY

Maya's first baby was easy, but just like all parenting, it wasn't without challenges. Laura's heel-prick test returned abnormalities revealing that she was born without a thyroid, a life-threatening condition that is easily and quickly rectified with synthetic thyroid hormones. Breastfeeding didn't come easily as it doesn't for most first time parents, and giving medication to an exclusive nurser was challenging, but temperament-wise, Laura was an easy baby. "She loved all the things babies are supposed to. She loved being swaddled, she loved sleeping on her back, she loved her swing. She was just a very easy baby."

"Then I had Cody, and I was like, 'I know what I'm doing. I have all the right stuff, and I know how to do all the right things.'"

"From the moment she came out, she did not stop screaming. 24/7 screaming. She hated everything. She wouldn't take a pacifier. Hated to be put down. Hated to be swaddled."

Maya knew something was wrong, but the pediatrician said she would grow out of it and that she just had colic. The only way for her to not be screaming was in the Rock 'n Play, an inclined rocker that has since been recalled, or with Maya standing upright with Cody in a baby carrier. "This sounds horrible, but I understood why people would want to shake their babies. I had a two-year-old, and every time I put Cody in the car seat, the swing, she would throw up. I couldn't do anything. I did not have postpartum depression, but I felt like, 'What is this creature that came into my life and ruined it.'"

At Cody's two-month appointment, Maya set her baby down for the exam and her pediatrician was finally able to see the level of reflux they were dealing with. While some babies don't experience any pain with reflux, it was very obvious that Cody did. They started medication, and after a few days, a new baby emerged. "It was night and day. She went from being so miserable to being so happy."

WEEKS SIX TO TWELVE

FOR BREAST-FED BABIES: 6–10 feeds in 24 hours, but at more regular intervals
FOR BOTTLE-FED BABIES: 6–10 (3–4 oz) bottles in 24 hours, but at more regular intervals

Prepare for the great wake up! Before six weeks, babies are so immature that if they are fed and comfortable, they will always fall right back to sleep. Between six and twelve weeks, sleepy newborns begin to mature enough to need help falling asleep. As babies need more active help sleeping enough, many parents worry that their baby isn't eating enough or something else is terribly wrong with feeding. However, if you are aware of tiredness cues, you can start to establish a more predictable sleeping and eating rhythm.

This phase of babyhood is hard, it is the peak of crying for newborn-hood. Resources like The Period of Purple Crying can offer some support during this time, you should also reach out to family and community for help. But at the end of the day, this is often period of parental desperation. Babies just cry a lot during this stretch. It is a huge developmental milestone, and it is gruelling. Just another one of those beautiful moments in parenting when you want to get it right and have very little control. The one thing you can control is trying, but not necessarily always succeeding, to help your baby get enough sleep.

If you gave birth, at six weeks, you will also likely have an appointment with your midwife or OB-GYN. Part of this visit is to clear you for sex and talk about contraception. I have met a few birthing people who were thrilled to be off pelvic rest, but most of us are still far from ready for this activity. That is fine. If you are nursing and have the kind of sex that can accidentally make new humans, it is worth asking your provider about contraceptives that don't impact milk supply.

TIREDNESS CUES AND ACTIVE SOOTHING

At some point between six and eight weeks, babies seem to wake all the way up and lose the ability to simply fall back asleep on their own. Your perfect "good sleeper" turns into a pterodactyl of hungry rage. As a baby's nervous system matures, it hits an awkward period when they still need to sleep basically all of the time, but it doesn't come easily to them. These moments of overtiredness can lead babies to cry much more and parents to think their baby must be starving, have an allergy, or be in some other kind of distress. Try to take a step back and notice if you baby is still eating well throughout the day and if they might just be having trouble getting enough sleep.

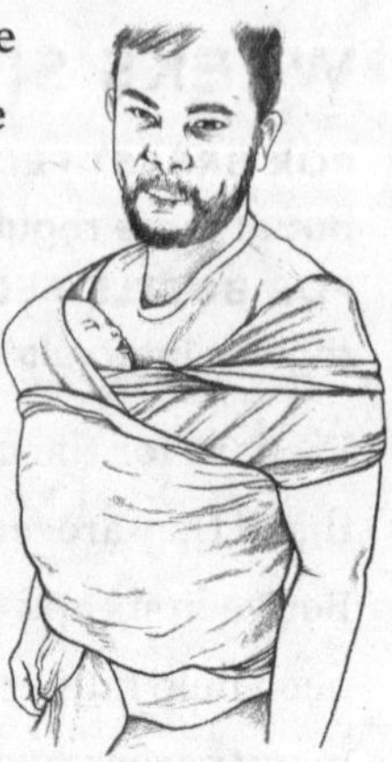

Baby's sleep cycles are the rhythm of happily awake and back into sleep that they need to stay content and do the very hard work of brain development. At this age, most babies can be happily awake for no more than ninety minutes (including eating) and then they will need a nap. They will then sleep for around forty-five minutes before coming into light sleep or even waking up. You can try to lull them into a second sleep cycle, which may last up to sixty minutes before they are ready to eat again. Some babies are naturally better at stitching these cycles together and consolidating sleep. People call these "easy babies," and honestly, it's just luck of the draw.

I liken this to being on a very long international flight. In coach. You are so tired, but you cannot sleep. The upright seat, the noise, the lights, the unfamiliar environment are all getting on your nerves. So, you yourself may start drinking or just slowly get less and less happy and more and more cranky. Imagine a kind attendant walked up to you just as you were shifting in your seat and said, *Oh hello, you seem tired, can I escort you to first class? Where we have a fluffy down comforter, a bed that lies flat, and earplugs?* You would say yes and settle into a big rest.

While many parents are in an all-out sprint to get to self-soothing and independent all-night sleep for their babies, that just isn't biologically normal for human babies. You can begin slowly working on some of those foundational sleep skills after twelve weeks, but for now, your only job is to notice tiredness cues and help your baby get to sleep.

So, how do you know when to escort your baby to first class? Begin by looking at their tiredness cues.

Early tiredness cues

- Looking away when you try to make eye contact
- Staring at high-contrast objects, like a fan or shadow
- Sneezing
- Hiccups

Late tiredness cues

- Arching
- Reflux (One of many possible causes. In this case a kid who rarely has reflux may have some when overtired.)
- Crying

It's a good idea to soothe a tired baby to sleep, and you can absolutely do this with feeding. You can also use tools like bouncing, swaddling, shushing, pacifiers, and a walk in a carrier to help your baby settle. You will know they are in a deep enough sleep to set down when their breathing gets slow and regular and they have noodle arms.

The longer they are awake, the harder it is to get them to sleep, and the less they will sleep overall. Confusingly, more daytime sleep equals more nighttime sleep.

Try to help your baby stay awake for a full feeding, then check the clock: If you are approaching that ninety-minute mark, go right into soothing. If your baby ate quickly and you have time, try some tummy time or play, but look out for those early tiredness cues and start sleep soothing when you see them.

Soothing tools

Responding to your baby's cues with the right tools helps build better communication.

SUCKING

Bottle feeding. Your baby may fall asleep drinking a bottle. That is fine at this age. After twelve weeks, take a look at this habit and decide if you are happy with it, or if you would like to wean onto a different sleep association.

Nursing. If you have no nipple damage, your baby has had a full feeding, and you don't need a shower, it is perfectly okay to let your baby nap/fall asleep with a nipple in their mouth. After twelve weeks, take a look at this habit and decide if you are happy with it, or if you would like to wean onto a different sleep association.

Pacifiers. Pacifiers are an essential tool. I do not recommend them before two weeks because they can hide feeding cues. After you are well-versed in what a full feeding looks like for your baby and how to know if your baby is hungry: pacify away.

WHITE NOISE

Babies like a continuous soundscape to sleep. They do not like harsh noises in silence. Shushing with your voice, a vacuum cleaner, or a white noise machine can help. It can also muffle sharp sounds like dogs barking or toddlers yelling.

HOLDING OR WEARING

Babies like to be snug. Wearing a baby in a carrier is a great way to get babies to sleep and still have hands free.

> Co-parents! Many non-nursing co-parents can find it hard to know their place in parenting. By mastering the nonfeeding soothing techniques, you can swoop in and give your partner a break, as well as teach your baby some nonfeeding soothing skills that will build sleep skills down the road. You can also use these tools to soothe a frustrated or hangry baby so they can calm down enough to try eating again. Talk to other parents to get their tips, find chunks of the day when you can be fully responsible for soothing, and give your partner a large break. Wearing a baby on a walk is a particularly good way to get some fresh air and give your partner time to rest.

You may find that during the first few days you try to get your baby to sleep a full ninety minutes to three hours between feedings at this age, you are holding or soothing them the entire nap to help connect their sleep cycles. This is normal and should get easier as your baby is less and less overtired. Eventually, they will get better at napping on their own and stretching their happily awake times after around eight weeks. This period of time can feel extremely overwhelming. It is absolutely exhausting to be needed so much. To sit, holding your baby, staring at that one spot on the wall you missed when repainting that you can't possibly fix because you are always and will always be holding a baby. I promise, the days of less crying are around the corner. Like most of parenting, this is just a phase.

If your baby seems to cry excessively beyond the normal week or two between weeks six and eight, your baby may be experiencing what is nebulously called colic (page 221).

SUPPLEMENTATION AND STARTING MIXED FEEDING

If you are wanting to combine nursing and formula feeding and haven't already, this is a good time. Milk production is more stable after six weeks and will be less dramatically impacted by skipping a feeding here and there while someone offers a bottle you did not make with your body.

You can also try exploring your body and your production without as much risk of production dropping or jumping up. That is to say that if you are away from your baby for longer stretches, you don't need to match up expression to the times when your baby eats, and you can instead see how your body responds to waiting for longer and longer stretches between expressing.

For instance, you may find that at the two-hour mark, you are able to pump 2 ounces, but at the three-hour mark, you are making 2.5, and at the four-hour mark you make 2.75. That slowdown or diminishing return tells us that your production edge is closer to the two-hour mark and to maintain your level of production, you should feed or express every two hours. You may instead find that at the two-hour mark, you make 2 ounces, at the three-hour mark, you make 3 ounces, at the four-hour mark you make

4 ounces, but at the five-hour mark, you make 4.5. That tells you that your edge is around the four-hour mark, and consistently going beyond that will start to impact overall production. Begin by incrementally going a little longer (at the same time of day if possible) and writing down how much you expressed and how long it was since the last feed/expression. This will start to give you some clues about your milk-storage capacity (page 236).

BOTTLE REFUSAL

After six weeks, some babies who haven't been introduced to bottles or are out of practice can be resistant to taking bottles. This can feel frustrating and scary, especially if a return to work is looming.

Try my "bottle boot camp" method

Start with a very warm bottle: while young babies or babies who are used to bottles may not worry about bottle temperature, the goal of bottle boot camp is to make bottle feeding as intriguing as possible. I call this bottle boot camp because working on bottle skills can take a lot of care and attention and may mess with your regular schedule. I recommend taking a weekend and approaching it like potty training: clear your schedule, ask for help, and really dedicate yourself to the task. If after a weekend of thoughtfully working on it, your baby still won't take a bottle, call in a professional to assess their sucking skills.

Start with a very warm bottle with about an ounce of milk in it. This smaller bottle will help keep pressure low about waste.

Watch your baby's nap for the light sleep phase. This looks like fluttering eyelids or a bit of wiggling around. Without lifting or otherwise disturbing your baby, gently touch their lips with the bottle, and wait for a response. If they stick their tongue out or open their mouth, that's your cue to slip the bottle into their mouth and let their sleepy suck reflex do the work.

If this worked, try again at the next few naps. Once this has worked at several light awake stages, you can start to try and offer a bottle to them when they are more and more awake.

If your baby refuses the bottle, leave it at room temperature and try again at the next feeding. This takes a lot of patience. While conventional wisdom says that the nursing parent can't even be in the same country as their baby while they are being offered a bottle, I find that what matters more is that the caregiver with the most bandwidth and patience in that moment offers a bottle.

Other tips and tricks to handle bottle refusal

DON'T TRY TO BOTTLE FEED A HUNGRY BABY

Bottle feeding is a different skill from nursing. This refusal is often related to the difficulty of learning a new way to eat. Most people don't learn very well when they are hangry. Try offering a bottle an hour after nursing, when your baby has eaten but is peckish. Babies will not get so hungry that they will just take a bottle. That would be entirely too logical, and that's not how babies operate.

OFFER A NO-PRESSURE BOTTLE

Start with a baby who is in their quiet, happy awake state. Tap the bottle nipple on their hand, then arm, then shoulder, then cheek, then lips. Just casually booping like a little game. Imagine someone comes out of nowhere and shoves a spoon of chili in your mouth. That would be pretty jarring. We tend to be protective about what goes into our mouths. Going slow can help babies not feel overwhelmed.

OFFER DIFFERENT SENSORY INPUT

Some of us study best with loud music; some of us need complete silence. Babies are people, too. Experiment with different amounts and kinds of sensory input. Offer a bottle in a dark, silent room. Or a dark room with lots of white noise. Or a bowling alley or kid's birthday party. Try swaddled and hugged close while bouncing on a yoga ball. Follow your intuition and your baby's cues to the right combo of sensory input for your baby.

WHAT ABOUT ALL THAT PACED BOTTLE FEEDING STUFF?

This can wait. Once your baby is used to bottles and has been reliably taking them for a week or two, then you can begin using those paced bottle techniques to continue developing their skills. Bottle refusers need us to make it as easy as possible at first and then build up skills gradually.

ALLERGIES OR INTOLERANCES: FORMULA

A few weeks into formula feeding, if your baby has rashes, constipation, diarrhea, or seems uncomfortable, it might be worth trying a formula switch. There's more on diagnosing the issue, as well as how to switch on page 146.

ALLERGIES OR INTOLERANCES: BREASTFEEDING

The most common trigger for allergies in food is protein. Protein from our food can migrate into milk and cause an allergic reaction in your baby. About three percent of babies have a cow's dairy allergy. Allergies are generally diagnosed by significant skin rashes and blood in the stool. Extremely stinky poop can also be an indicator. In families that have a genetic predisposition to allergies, it is worth keeping an eye on your baby for allergies, even when exclusively feeding them your milk. For instance, if celiac runs in the family, it may be recommended that the nursing parent stay away from gluten while nursing. While most babies aren't sensitive enough to allergens to react to them in milk, some babies are. The gluten proteins that cause a celiac reaction can impact nursing babies, as can soy or dairy, and in some even rarer cases, things like shellfish. All of these elimination diets should be conducted under the advice of a gastroenterologist (GI doctor) or allergist, because they can give you the most current recommendations on reintroducing these foods and how to introduce solids.

Elimination diets

Some babies are not allergic to these proteins but have trouble digesting them. The difficulty in identifying this kind of intolerance is that the symptoms can be traced to many causes. Ask your pediatrician for a referral to a gastroenterologist who can help you parse out these differences.

Once sure you've ruled out other causes, you may consider an elimination diet for intolerances.

Parenthood is hard enough, so I wouldn't recommend going to this option first. It can take up to two weeks for some proteins to leave your milk, so you won't get reliable feedback on this very quickly. Most people undertaking an elimination diet start by eliminating dairy, soy, and corn. This can be really difficult to do while eating enough and making food for your baby. Taking this on with a plan, go to the store and buy lots of food you can eat, and after two weeks, note if you are seeing a decrease in your baby's symptoms.

What about cabbage and beans? There is no real evidence that eating farty foods yourself means your baby will have gas. Babies cry. If your baby cries excessively (see page 221) talk to your doctor about possible causes. As for my recommendation: If there are no clear risk factors for allergies, eat what you like and plenty of it. There is no need for a special diet while nursing. I raise this glass of rosé and plate of soft cheeses to you. Cheers.

PREBIOTICS AND PROBIOTICS

Your baby's microbiome is a complex ecosystem of bacteria that live on their skin, in their gut, in their sinuses. This ecosystem helps keep our bodies heathy and does a lot of our immunity and digestion. It is extremely important and still mostly a mystery. Like outer space.

What we do know

PREBIOTICS

These are nutrients that feed our biome. Human milk contains tons of human milk oligosaccharides (or HMOs), and they differ from person to person. Your baby cannot digest them; they are food you make for your baby's bacteria, not your baby. Since these carbohydrates are so variable and complex, we cannot easily replicate them in formula. Luckily, one of the main HMOs is lactose, which is in many infant formulas. As prebiotics are tested and better understood, they will make their way into health recommendations for nursing parents and infant formula alike.

PROBIOTICS

Probiotics are the bacteria themselves. These bacteria can be sensitive to stress, get wiped out by antibiotics, or be different based on birth style.

We don't understand these changes and their impacts well enough to say that any of this is bad, but we do know that sometimes boosting the probiotics you ingest can help settle some digestive or skin issues you may be seeing.

If your baby has "colicky" digestion (a.k.a. painful gas, difficulty pooping, a seemingly upset tummy), you may want to add more prebiotics and probiotics to their diet to help out.

Many baby probiotics are on the market, and I recommend getting them separately rather than hunting down an infant formula that contains them.

When adding pro and prebiotics, go slow. Our digestion doesn't appreciate abrupt changes. So, talk to your pediatrician about the correct dosage for your baby. Spread that dose throughout the day. Plan to work up to a full recommended dose over the course of two weeks or so.

Here we are, at the end of the fourth trimester. Your tiny, underdeveloped baby is now ready to work on a whole new world of development. Feedings should have gotten faster and more consolidated. Your baby can be awake for longer stretches and interact more. You've learned how to tell if your baby is overtired and how to get them to sleep. You've hopefully found a nursing routine or formula that works well for you, maybe both. Keep exploring together. You might even be getting ready to leave the house for more than a doctor's appointment. When I worked as a postpartum doula, I loved this transition. This was when I worked myself out of a job and watched my cocooned little family start to blossom into its own unit.

My hope is that you are starting to see yourselves in your new little family unit. That your baby's personality is emerging to you, and that you are finding rhythms that work for you. Did you find some community with other people who are sharing your new roles? Lean into those relationships as you start to venture more into a big, wide world.

CHAPTER 10

LIFE BEYOND THE NEWBORN STAGE (TWELVE WEEKS TO SIX MONTHS)

FOR BREAST-FED BABIES: 6–10 feeds per 24 hours, but at more regular intervals

FOR BOTTLE-FED BABIES: 6–10 feeds; some may be taking fewer, larger bottles, such as 6 6-ounce bottles per 24 hours. Talk to your baby's doctor if your baby is eating well over 32 ounces per day.

Welcome to your new alert and distracted baby. You can no longer hold an iced coffee without little hands reaching to explore it. You'll notice that, suddenly, your baby is distracted by everything. It's not uncommon for babies to have a lot of trouble focusing on eating because the dog, a sibling, a shadow is just too interesting. You'll also notice that no cup or sandwich is safe. As babies get developmentally ready to start eating solid foods, they become very interested in your dining habits. Get ready for a lot of face grabbing and . . . commonly, a pretty big sleep regression. We will also talk about excessive crying and colic in this section. As we leave the newborn hood, if your baby still seems uncomfortable or difficult to soothe there may be more going on.

SCHEDULES

As your baby approaches twelve weeks, you may find that rhythms and schedules start to emerge for you. Ideally, this is based around your baby's happy awake times. Here is a common flow of a day:

5:00 a.m.: Feeding

5:30 a.m.: Back to sleep

7:00 a.m.: Up for the day, feeding

7:30 a.m.: Happy playtime; parent eats breakfast and pumps if pumping to offer bottles

8:30 a.m.: Nap

10:00 a.m.: Feeding

11:30 a.m.: Nap

1:00 p.m.: Feeding

2:30 p.m.: Nap

4:00 p.m.: Feeding

5:30–9:00 p.m.: Cluster feeding, nap fighting, bath time

9:00 p.m.: Big sleep

1:00 a.m.: Feeding, back to sleep.

You'll notice this is not a perfect schedule with a bunch of directions; it is a loose imaging of the rhythm a lot of babies fall into. Follow your baby's own hungry, awake, asleep cycles and nudge to make sure they get enough daytime naps.

Is it wrong to let the baby snack? Nope. You get to feed your baby how you choose. If you want to keep your baby fully on demand, that is just fine. If your baby is bottle-fed, you'll want to keep an eye on their weight for overfeeding and switch to a pacifier for soothing if overfeeding is a concern.

CRYING AND COMMUNICATION

As you may be learning from all the cues laid out here, crying is a late cue of a lot of things. Unfortunately, there will be times where you cannot decode the early cues or simply cannot get to your baby in time. Your baby will cry. You know it is part of the territory with babies, but nothing can prepare you for the full mental exhaustion/empathy/heartbreak/rage/desire to run away that is a baby crying. Some babies cry a lot (this is called *colic,* which I'll explain later in this chapter), but all babies cry. Here are some ways to cope.

Take breaks or your baby will break you

As horrible as it sounds, at some point or another, most of us feel the impulse to shake our babies. You aren't a bad person, and you aren't alone. If you feel yourself getting overwhelmed by crying, you can and should take a break. Set a timer for ten minutes and set your baby down in a safe place (blanket on the floor in a room with no other kids or pets, or in a crib) and walk away.

Go outside and breathe. Hide in the pantry and eat a snack. Take a drink of water. Go pee. Cry. Call a friend. Scream. Or all of the above. All good parents have done this. Your baby can cry for alone ten minutes and be absolutely fine.

When you are ready, come back and try some soothing techniques. If you get overwhelmed again, it is okay to take another break. If you are trapped in a cycle, call in help if you can.

Step in if you see a parent getting overwhelmed. No need to remark on the situation, which can trigger a shame spiral. Just pour a glass of water and say, "Hey, let me take that baby for a minute. I poured you a glass of water. We'll be back in a little bit." Step outside or into another room with baby and let that parent have a minute to rebalance.

Troubleshooting excessive crying

COLIC

What exactly is colic? Your guess is as good as mine. This diagnosis refers to a total amount of crying. This is a symptom, not a cause. It is defined as more than three hours of crying daily for more than three days per week. Most practitioners think that it probably relates back to a baby's gut. Over history, some babies have just cried more than others. Humans have done all kinds of things to help colicky babies and their parents, most notably giving them opium and alcohol, which did help them sleep but is no longer recommended for reasons that I hope are obvious. Babies hit the peak of their crying around six to eight weeks, so if you have a baby who already cries a lot, this is a time when you are desperate for solutions. This kind of crying can be caused by digestive discomfort, sensory dysregulation, or pain that isn't understood yet.

FOREMILK/HINDMILK IMBALANCE

As we discussed on page 134, high milk supply can cause an imbalance that is really uncomfortable for babies. This can cause babies to have a painful upset stomach. The best clue is bright-green mucussy poop. If that's the case, try some strategies to bring down production on page 133.

GUT OVERGROWTH/FOOD SENSITIVITY

Some people have an overgrowth of a certain bacteria that reacts to certain food. Basically, you are feeding a colony of bacteria, and as they digest that food, they give off gas that uncomfortably fills the large intestine. Signs of this would be painful gas, a distended stomach, or stinky gas/poop accompanying the crying.

TONGUE-TIE

Babies who swallow air or have tired muscles due to a tongue-tie may cry more than other babies. You should have a colicky baby assessed for a tie if their shoulders often seem hunched, their tongue sits low in their mouth when crying, or they have a lot of burps.

GUT RESTRICTION

Just as bones and muscles can get cramped in the development or birth process, so can guts. Our squishy intestines can get kinked, making it hard to pass gas or poop. If your baby has painful gas but it does not smell, you may want to see an infant bodyworker (page 57) about alignment.

Nondigestive causes of excessive crying

CHRONIC OVERTIREDNESS

Some babies have a particularly hard time settling into frequent naps. If your baby cries a lot and doesn't seem to sleep much (babies should sleep about eighteen hours per day), try using some of the sleep strategies on page 209 to catch early tiredness cues and help your baby sleep.

UNDERREGULATED NERVOUS SYSTEM

Some babies have a hard time regulating their sensory system and need more or less input than other people. Babies who are sensory seeking do best with lots of noise, bouncing, car rides, and sucking. Babies who are sensory avoidant like white noise or quiet, being held still, and being laid down by themselves. It can be very challenging to figure out what your baby's sensory needs are, but once you understand them, you can use this to help them regulate. If you suspect your baby falls in this category, an occupational therapist may be able to help.

PERSONALITY

Some babies just need a lot of hands-on care and cry a lot. And it's hard. These are usually the coolest kids, but the hardest babies. Get yourself as much help as you can. It can be hard to hand off a crying baby, but people who have slept through the night tend to mind crying a lot less, and a shower and a walk around the block can really help you cope with these hard days.

LOWER DIGESTION

After the stomach, we begin the second half of digestion. This is where the important gut flora is and where the absorption of nutrients and water happens. The first stop on this journey is the small intestine. This is where the globs of fat and sugar in milk get moved through the walls of the gut into the bloodstream to be used for energy or stored.

Next stop is the large intestine. This is where water is absorbed from what was once milk and where the microbiome mostly lives and is fed. This last bit of digestion is so important to health in ways we don't even know about yet, but here are a few fun facts we do know:

- Babies start developing a microbiome in utero by swallowing amniotic fluid. It continues to change until around six months after birth, when they start eating solid food and the guts of adults and babies look just about the same, but they tend to resemble that of other members of their family.
- The bacteria in the lower intestine make vitamin K. Vitamin K is a very important part of making blood clot. Newborns are given vitamin K at birth to prevent brain bleeds because they don't have a developed enough gut to make it on their own.
- About 70 percent of our immune system lives in our gut. When a baby drinks human milk, the antibodies and immune cells in the milk reside in the gut and protect against viruses and infection until babies are old

enough to make their own. Formula-fed babies work with the gut flora they make on their own or have from pregnancy and birth.

The large intestine is where farts are made. If you have a baby who is very gassy, it has one of two causes. Air that is swallowed as part of a messy suck and not burped in the first half of eating will come out down here in the second half of digestion. This is by far the more uncomfortable way to get air out. So, babies who don't have other signs of an allergy should be burped rigorously while you get to the bottom of why they are swallowing air in the first place. If a baby has gas that smells, it is an indicator that their microbiome is making gas. Gas is usually the result of an intolerance, a part of food your baby can't digest, or an overgrowth of bacteria. While a cow's milk allergy might cause reflux, rashes, or even trouble breathing, a cow dairy sensitivity will cause bloating and smelly gas. Both are fairly uncommon (about 2–3 percent of babies under one year) but can lead to discomfort and "colic."

CURIOUS BABIES

The hallmark of this period of development and feeding is distraction. As your baby gains more control over their body, they want to explore it. Suddenly, every little noise and light must be investigated. This is a very exciting time, but for feeding, it can also be frustrating. It may be an option to do some or all feedings in a few quiet locations. White noise and predictability can help very distractible eaters. For most people, this isn't really an option. Siblings, the dog, the phone will all just be things that need tending to. Unfortunately, there is really no magic solution for this; it is just how development goes. If you are nursing, know that you get a say in things. If it is just too frustrating to nurse in these moments, or painful from your baby popping on and off, you have the choice to stop and try again later, to wean, or to offer a bottle.

It's fairly common for babies to just get good at managing their nursing at this point. It is a good time to experiment with new positions, like sitting up while nursing or to try to eliminate the need for a nipple shield, if you would like to. To do this, you can either offer a non-shielded latch between typical feeding times, when your baby is less hungry, or start nursing with the shield and remove it part way through. Try to be open and experimental about it.

Your baby may do fewer, larger feedings at this age, or do the same number but cluster them more to the daytime. Though your baby may not be ready to sleep through the night yet, these longer stretches at night without feeding can start to decrease your supply.

Here is a loose nighttime schedule for a baby this age—the schedule I see most parents do to maintain production:

Between 7:00 and 8:00 p.m.: Nurse/pump a bottle before the baby goes to bed.

Between 10:00 and 11:00 p.m.: Dream feed or night pump to express before parent goes to bed.

4:00–6:00 a.m.: Nurse and then settle down for another snooze.

9:00 a.m.: Nurse or pump.

After 9:00 a.m.: Whatever daytime feeding/expressing looks like for you during the day.

If you have a longer storage time or less of a need/desire to maintain your production level, you can drop any of the above nursings/expressions and be just fine.

FOUR-MONTH SLEEP REGRESSION

As babies do all of these exciting brain developments, they also sometimes just forget how to sleep, a.k.a. go through a four-month sleep regression. This is usually short-lived, so just try to survive it. You might notice that your baby eats a lot more during this regression or eats much more at night because they are distracted during the day.

HOW TO GET THROUGH A NURSING STRIKE

Some babies will have bouts of refusing to nurse. This is common and usually lasts a few hours or days. At this age, nursing strikes are often brought on by illness or a new neurological development. When babies develop new social awareness, they are often very distractible or are exploring the emotional response of refusing to nurse. The key to moving through a nursing strike regardless of the cause is to casually wait it out. Use pumping or hand expression to maintain supply and continue to offer nursing in a low-pressure way. Try not to react strongly to a refusal. It can also help to go to a gathering where other people will be nursing. Sometimes seeing other babies nursing with their parents kickstarts your baby to go back to it.

During a strike, you should offer pumped milk or formula in other ways (bottles, open cups, or straws) and continue to offer nursing.

If a strike lasts more than two weeks, your baby may have chosen to wean, and you can begin the process of expressing less to gradually bring down your milk production.

BOTTLE NIPPLES

You may have noticed that bottle nipples have sizes on them, starting with preemie or slow flow and going up to around the number 4. These numbers mark the width of the hole that milk comes out of. You do not need to ever increase or "graduate" to the next size. The goal is to keep resistance high so that babies have to use their mouth muscles to draw milk out, and eventually eat solids and speak. If your baby is starting to refuse bottles or is clustering larger bottles to the day and night weaning, you may want to go up in size and see if bottles become less frustrating.

MILK-MAKING AND MENSTRUATION

People return to menstruating after pregnancy at different rates, but if you are lactating, it commonly follows longer stretches between nursing or expressing. When you do return to menstruating, it can often add another variable to your milk production. When your progesterone spikes, it can temporarily dip production. This isn't usually very noticeable when nursing, because your baby would just eat more often or longer. It is noticeable when pumping because you are looking at volume numbers. If you are worried about the dip, you can add an extra pumping during that time and then drop it when that phase of your cycle is over.

FEEDING AND SLEEP TRAINING

This age brings a transition in how babies sleep, or more specifically, how they self-soothe. If a baby is gaining weight well between four and six months, your pediatrician will clear you to begin whatever sleep training works for your family if desired. During this period this kind of sleep learning looks like setting babies down more and more awake to soothe themselves to sleep. That doesn't mean your baby is ready to sleep through the night, but they may be ready to start building those skills.

Sleep training is its own extremely personal and controversial topic, but since we like choices in this family, I will begin by saying this: You get to choose what is right for your family. Sleep training may be what you need to work on to maintain a stable mood. It is also completely fine to stay at the other end of the spectrum and feed your baby through the night and based on cues for as long as you would like. I have seen points all along this spectrum work great for families, just like all the points along a spectrum of exclusive nursing to exclusive bottle feeding.

In my experience, these choices always have trade-offs. I have noticed in my years in the field that there is a gradient of flexibility to predictability. Babies who eat on demand and sleep with their parents (these two things don't always go together, nor do they have to) are very flexible but not very predictable. Their feeding and sleep association is their parents, so they can happily do those things, as long as those tools are there. On the other end of the spectrum, babies who eat and sleep on a very specific schedule in specific locations are very predictable but not very flexible. Sometimes where you are on this spectrum is related to your baby's temperament; sometimes it is based on family needs.

It is possible to start sleep training between four and six months, and there are two key elements to this process. Sleep training is teaching a baby to self soothe and combine sleep cycles (this can be done in many ways) and night weaning, which is stretching out the length of time your baby goes without eating in the night and clustering their calorie intake in the day. These two things are often done together, but they are independent variables. You can teach a baby to soothe and sleep without food and still feed them in the night if they are hungry. You would just have them fall back to sleep in a way that didn't involve eating.

If you are exclusively using formula or donor milk, there is only one variable to adjust as you figure out a sleep pattern that works for you: your baby. If your baby is gaining weight well, tolerates fewer larger feedings, and your pediatrician gives you the sign-off, you can adjust sleep however suits you, including full night weaning.

If you are nursing or pumping in the night, you have two variables: your baby and your body. Take a second to review the section about milk storage versus production on page 236. If your milk storage is such that your baby can nurse/drink bottles throughout the day and get enough to eat, then night weaning without pumping may work great for you. If your storage capacity is shorter than the time you would like to be asleep, sleeping through without nursing or pumping will decrease your overall supply. I think this is a reasonable trade-off in a world where you are expected to be remarkably smart and human soon after you have a baby, but for some people, this possible drop in production feels really scary. If that's true for you, decide what feels easiest in the night: pumping or nursing. If you choose nursing, you can either nurse your baby back to sleep, or nurse them and use other soothing for them to fall back asleep, because night weaning and sleep training are different things.

WAYS TO SLEEP TRAIN WHILE MAINTAINING PRODUCTION

If you want to have it both ways, here are a few ideas of how to maintain more milk production and still teach your baby to sleep through the night.

Night pumping

Some people find waking up to pump less disruptive than waking up with a baby. You can pump right before bed and set an alarm to pump when you have hit your max storage in the night.

Night nursing

Some people just don't find it that disruptive to nurse at night. If you don't, then carry on.

Lots of babies like to fall asleep sucking. When we come up into a light sleep and roll over, fluff out pillow, etc., we expect to fall asleep again in the same way we did last time. Imagine you feel asleep cozy in your bed and woke up in the middle of the night in the middle of the kitchen floor. You would not just fall back asleep. This is how babies feel when they fall asleep eating and then wake up one sleep cycle later with nothing to suck on. If consolidating sleep stretches and self-soothing are important to you, you will need to break that association by having your baby fall asleep while not eating. This can be done gradually.

This is to say that babies who have an eating association with sleep tend to wake more frequently than babies who don't. This is biologically normal and completely fine. It may or may not fit into your life routine.

If you feel like independent sleep is important to your family's wellbeing, you can make changes.

I do not offer any of this to say that babies should or have to sleep through the night at this or any age. I offer it because many parents enter sleep teaching without knowing how it may impact feeding and milk production. This is a risk-benefit calculation. If you need sleep and are comfortable with your milk supply going down overall, that self-knowledge will guide your choices. If your milk production is extremely important to you and waking up at night to maintain it suits you, then that's all the information you need.

RETURNING TO WORK AND FEEDING IN PUBLIC

By now, you and your baby should be well acquainted and ready to start venturing into the world. But in the US, this often means it is time to return to working, which can be complicated. Many of us are happy to rediscover our roles at work and in other parts of our life, but this time can also feel abrupt, like being pushed out of the nest into a harsh new reality. The

MICHELLE'S STORY

Michelle started parenting with four hundred ounces of pumped milk in the freezer and a body that had big supply reserves. This is because Michelle had induced lactation via pumping while planning for her open adoption. With the permission of her daughter's birth mother, she used hormones and pumping to start lactating and nursed her baby for three years, using bottles and formula when they were out and about. That part of their experience was pretty simple.

Sleep was another story. "It was the unpredictability that made my anxiety so bad. I needed to lay my head on the pillow knowing if I would wake up one time or five. If I would be awake for five minutes or two hours." While her wife had a much easier time with the night wakings, it was destroying Michelle's mental health. Michelle set out to try to get her baby to fall asleep independently as the best choice for their family, but every time she caved and nursed her baby to sleep, she felt like a failure. She started to learn from sleep consultants how to build a more consistent sleep routine and to help her daughter self-soothe by checking on her at regular intervals to give everyone more predictability. Eventually, Michelle knew she would be able to sleep through the night and her mood improved immeasurably. It wasn't a linear path, but they eventually got there. She went on from that experience to become a sleep consultant, helping families find the right blend of approaches to meet their needs. Here's the system she advises as the Baby Sleep Engineer:

At four to six months, your baby can start to learn to put themselves to sleep. This can be done with a range of tools, from gradually setting your baby down more and more awake to full extinction, where you set down a fully awake baby and let them move through self-soothing to sleep (usually through crying) until they are asleep. Start by moving the last feeding before bedtime away from the bedtime routine. Place it before books and jammies in the schedule so that it isn't a big part of their sleep association. Bedtime is set by most American sleep consultants at 7:00 p.m. If you are worried about your milk production dropping from not draining, or you need more milk for the next day, add a pumping session before you go to bed. Soothe or don't (whatever way corresponds to your sleep plan) without feeding until the first wake-up after midnight. At that wake-up, feed your baby and then let them soothe themselves, or soothe them yourself in other ways to get back to sleep. Offer the next feeding when they wake up for the day, after 6:00 a.m.

6:30 p.m.: Last feeding of the "day"
7:00 p.m.: Bedtime without eating
10:00 p.m.: Pump if nursing or pumping
12:01 a.m. or after: Nurse/bottle feed/pump
6:00 a.m. or after: Nurse/bottle feed/pump

demands of returning to work while your baby still doesn't sleep all night and needs a lot of care and perhaps food from your body are huge. I would even argue, unfair. Most people don't have much real choice around when and how to return to work.

RETURNING TO WORK AND PUMPING LOGISTICS

I have helped people who travel the world for international aid organizations, work from prisons as defense lawyers, and in offices with their own gorgeous lactation suites. I've known teachers who pumped during recess and dental hygienists who used in-bra pumps and pumped while cleaning teeth. We are diverse and have diverse workplaces.

First, let's think about where you will pump. You will gradually find out how often and when you need to pump, but in order to do that, we start with the where.

Start before you go on leave. Notify your employer that when you return to work, you intend to pump and will need adequate space and breaks to do so. Ask to see the space they have in mind and be as explicit as possible. Unfortunately, legal protections for pumping only extend to hourly employees. Generally speaking, though, employers want to keep employees and will do what they can if you are explicit about your needs. If your employer can't meet these needs, we have all learned during COVID shutdowns that most salaried jobs can be done from home, where there is a lot of private space to pump.

What to tell your employer you need

- A private space with a lockable door that is not used for another purpose such that you might be interrupted
- An outlet
- A sink
- Refrigeration for milk and pump part storage

The laws around this in the US are complicated, but most employers will work with you to find a good place, especially if you are clear about what are not acceptable options. For example, bathrooms, storage closets, and large meeting rooms without privacy and locks are not acceptable options. That being said, there are exceptions to every rule. The lawyer working in prisons had no good option besides the bathroom and was comfortable with her choice. She had a system for cleaning and setting up, using a passive-suction hand pump to minimize things that needed to be cleaned and brought with her on those occasions. If you work going from home to home doing pediatric therapy visits, like my daughter's speech therapist, then pumping in your car might just be the best spot for you.

If you work in an office, you should be able to take twenty- to thirty-minute breaks and use a room or office with a lock as many times as you need to pump. If your pump isn't rechargeable, you will need an outlet. While a sink is ideal, access to a fridge to hold pump parts and milk will work fine, but it needs to be a dedicated fridge or well-labeled specific area of the fridge that is only for your pumping use. This is all so specific that you may need to have a real conversation with your manager or HR department. If this is the first time they have addressed this need, it may require some collaboration. Try to open these conversations as soon as possible and be as specific as possible.

Some parents opt to have their children brought to them or go to their children, rather than pumping. This works particularly well if your child-care is located in your workplace.

Kim, a surgical physician assistant, would scrub out and meet her husband in the parking lot to nurse their baby. He took a step back from his work as a ship captain and was a stay-at-home dad. He would drive to the hospital between surgeries so Kim could nurse in the car. "It was just so much faster. I was so grateful to him for doing that."

If you are returning to school and your classes cannot be remote, talk to a guidance counselor about how to schedule classes around your needs, access to refrigeration, and campus pumping rooms.

Pack your pumping bag

What you need

- Hand towel
- Pump kit: flanges, tubing, membranes, bottles
- Extra-large Ziploc bags
- Cooler bag
- Extra bottles, milk storage bags, or large water bottle for milk transport
- Snack
- Water bottle for you
- If it's in your budget, a whole second kit of pump parts to leave at work, in case you forget a part of your pump kit

Daily schedule

- Pack up your clean and dry pump kit and put it in your bag with your pump and any other items you need.
- Use the principles of "body milk storage" (later in this section, page 236) to determine how many times you need to pump at work to maintain your production. This doesn't need to match up with your baby's eating schedule.
- At the end of the day, pack up your milk and put it in your cooler bag to take home. Remember that milk is fine at room temp for over eight hours, so you don't need to wash your pump parts during the day. Some people who have a fridge in their office keep their pump parts in there all week and bring them home on the weekend to wash.
- Wash and dry your pump kit (flanges, membranes, and bottles; not tubing).

PARTNERS

Processing milk is a great partner task. Especially if your co-parent is pumping, or doing drop-off and pickup, this is a good way to spread the work around. Set up a system that works for you and take ownership of it.

Bottle prep for daycare

Preparing milk to send with your baby to daycare will range from very informal to very strict depending on the setting. Keeping track of milk is important to the daycare for safety, and so these rules can be fairly strict.

Some rules you may encounter:

- No glass bottles
- Specifics on labeling
- Sending premixed bottles of formula
- No reuse of unfinished breast milk bottles

Preparing milk for daycare

You will need to establish how much your baby takes per feeding and pre-prepare the bottles for the day. Having good estimates on your baby's intake will help prevent waste or overfeeding.

The night before, you can process that day's pumped milk into bottles for the next day. If there is not enough, pull milk from the freezer to the fridge to thaw for the next day or prepare a formula bottle to make up the difference. Some families prefer to send a formula "buffer bottle" to prevent wasting pumped milk if their baby sometimes takes a little extra and sometimes doesn't.

If you are formula feeding, mix the formula together into bottles and refrigerate.

Apply labels with the date and name of your baby.

Occasionally, a mix up will happen and your baby may get a bottle intended for another baby of vice versa. This can be extremely stressful. Try to remain calm and speak to the other set of parents. If it was your milk given, you may need to drop by and replace that bottle.

If your baby was given milk for another child and does not have any food allergies, it should be fine. If they do have allergies, you will want the team to closely monitor them for the rest of the day.

From a disease or contamination perspective: people care deeply for their babies and are usually very careful not to consume anything dangerous or provide milk if they have a transmissible viral infection.

UNDERSTANDING SUPPLY AND STORAGE CAPACITY

When people talk about milk supply, they usually refer to having "high supply" or "low supply," meaning that they made more or less milk than their baby or babies needed. There is another detail to how people make milk that isn't captured in this. If your baby is nursing, it's fairly irrelevant; you feed them when they are hungry, and that's it. When you start to spend periods of time apart, you have a new milk-supply relationship with your fridge/pump. The goal of expressing milk while away is to replenish whatever your baby ate while you were apart. Many people do this by pumping at the intervals when they would ordinarily nurse, but depending on your storage capacity, this may be unnecessary.

Ready for a bit of a math problem? These three containers symbolize different people's milk storage.

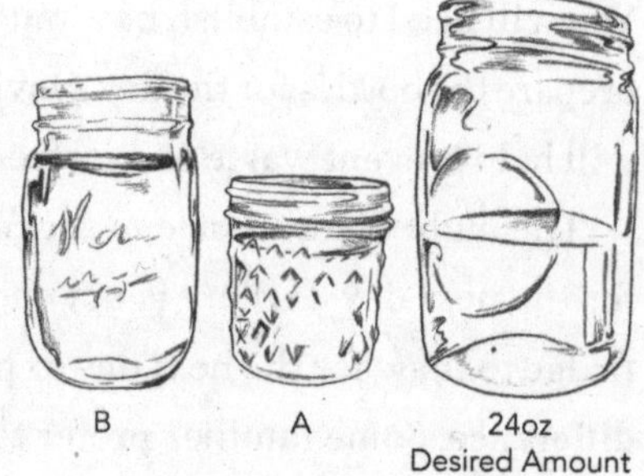

Now, we aren't talking about feedings here. This is purely about breast drainage. For some people it may take a few feeds to "drain" a breast (remember, milk-making is a perpetual motion machine, so breasts are never really empty). Let's imagine you are away from your baby and only expressing. In order for both these people to make twenty-four ounces to bring home for their baby, Person A, with the smaller cup, needs to refill more times to fill the twenty-four-ounce jar. That person will need to pump every few hours. After two hours, that person will feel uncomfortably full, and if they wait and pump every four hours, their cup will be full every time, and they will still only pump two ounces, leaving them with only twelve ounces to bring home. That's fine by me; that person might need work or sleep, but the difference will need to be made up with another food source, and it will gradually bring their production level down because their body is getting the signal that less milk is needed/wanted.

Person B has a bigger cup. They aren't better or cooler or stronger. They did not do a better job. This is just their biology. Bodies. Are. Different. This person can fill up and pump three times per day and make the twenty-four ounces needed to send home. Say that person decides to be extra decadent and get ten hours of sleep while away in a hotel room. They will wake up uncomfortably full and still only get eight ounces. Eight ounces or eight hours is their point of diminishing returns.

Another aspect of pumping at work that may be different for you is how long it takes. A standard fifteen-minute break doesn't capture the full picture of expressing milk. Here are a few things that can help make pumping at work go more smoothly, but how long your body takes to be well drained by a pump is a body-to-body difference.

- Wear easy pumping clothes: The less you have to undress and redress, the faster you will be able to pump. Wearing something with buttons down the front or wearing separates so you can pull a shirt up to your neck is great. You may also consider bras that double from regular bras into pumping bras. Having free hands is essential for multi-tasking, as well as for using your hands for massage while pumping, which helps you express more efficiently.
- Massage a bit before you pump: Go ahead and give your body a little skin-to-skin touch, maybe some big swoops or shakes of your chest to wake up the system. Hand express a little bit.
- While pumping, try to minimize stress and pain. If the email you have been dreading can wait, put it off. Remember that higher suction doesn't create better milk removal. It's the signal to your brain that has the biggest impact, so pumping should feel comfortable but effective. I want you to be able to say, "I feel that, but it doesn't hurt."
- Wash pump parts when the day is done, but wash your hands before every time you pump. Remember, pumping is food prep, so start the day with clean pump parts and keep some hand sanitizer in your bag. Ideally, you'll fully wash your hands before pumping, but hand sanitizer works great in a pinch. Your pump parts can go into a reusable wet bag, gallon plastic bag, or basin while you are at work. Assuming your workday is less than twelve hours and in a cool, clean place, you can wash everything when you get home

rather than every time you pump. If you are working on a construction site in the summer, for instance, try keeping parts in a cooler to use throughout the day.

- Use the milk-pooling technique: Instead of pumping into new bottles every time, empty milk into a larger water bottle. There are some amazing water bottles out there these days that hold a lot of liquid and keep it very temperature stable. Some even have a freezable core, so you don't need a refrigerator. You can add fresh milk to cool or room temperature milk and then put it in bottles for the next day when you get home and freeze anything leftover.

BOTTLE-FEEDING IN PUBLIC

The main challenge of bottle feeding in public is keeping milk cool in transit and warm for drinking, depending on your baby's preferences and how long you are out and about.

For pumped milk

Carry a cooler with bottles of milk, either pooled in an insulated water bottle or individually portioned into your feeding bottles. I find that soft freezable coolers work great. If your baby is picky about temperature, bring a separate insulated bottle full of hot water and a tumbler to warm bottles in.

If you will be out less than eight hours and the temperature is relatively cool, you can premake bottles so they are ready to go, but if it's hot out, keep them in a cooler bag.

For formula

Depending on the temperatures outside and how long you'll be out, you can premix a bottle of formula and take it with you. If it will be more than two hours or it's hot out, you'll want to keep water and formula separate. If your baby prefers bottles to be a specific temperature, you can fill a good vacuum-walled water bottle or thermos with the temperature of water you desire and then add it to a bottle when your baby is ready to eat. Then, bring a separate container with the desired number of scoops of formula in it and add to the baby bottle of water. Toss any mixed bottles if your baby doesn't finish them. Make sure that if you have powdered formula in a container in your bag as backup that you pull it out and use it at least every week so it's not sitting around at various temperatures, separated from its expiration date and lot number.

NURSING IN PUBLIC

In the early days, you may require a lot of pillows and a very specific environment to nurse. I recommend starting small by going to a friend's house or a parenting meetup where there are extra pillows and kind faces. As you and your baby have more practice, it'll get easier to leave the house.

In the US, you are legally allowed to nurse anywhere that you are allowed to be. For instance, if you aren't a platinum member of Delta you cannot nurse in the Sky Lounge. But if you are, go right ahead. Some people find it more comfortable personally to wear a cover to nurse. This should be for your comfort, not the comfort of others. Generally speaking, nursing isn't actually that exposing of an activity, unless your baby is over six months old and is constantly distracted and pops on and off, thus exposing you. Again, this is fine, but is based on your comfort.

If you need to lie back to nurse, you can tuck your bag into your chair at the small of your back to lean on, or use the recline of the passenger seat of your parked car.

How to nurse in a carrier

Another great way to nurse pretty privately in public is to do so in a carrier. This is mostly only an option for people after the twelve-week mark, because you and your baby are both just now getting good enough at nursing to get creative. The first time you attempt this, have help around. Someone to loosen and tighten straps is helpful.

In a wrapped carrier: Wrap your carrier a little more loosely than you would normally. When you put your baby in, angle them toward the side you are trying to nurse on. Adjust their lower body in the carrier and, standing or sitting, latch your baby. Once they are latched, you can pull up the rest of the carrier around them to secure them. As always, you need to be able to see your baby and make sure their airways are nice and clear.

Nursing in a soft-structured carrier: Put your baby on you as you would

normally. Then, loosen the waist strap to adjust your baby to the level of your chest. Loosen the arm strap on the side that you want to latch on, and use your arm on that side to hold your breast and latch. Once latched, you can tighten straps until you are both comfortable.

There is a lot we don't have control over in raising babies. When you add work and not having control of your schedule into the mix, things get even more difficult. Remember, you are more than how you feed your baby. Most of us feel like we are treading water at this point. Your healthy mood, sleep needs, work schedule, or family demands may dictate how often it is reasonable to take the time to express. That may mean that you are supplementing more (with formula, donor milk, or your freezer stash), and that is fine by me. It can feel anxiety-inducing to watch your production decrease, but try to remember, there is no research that says it is dangerous to supplement, and that abundance is spreading to other parts of your life. The abundance you once had in milk transforms to an abundance of sleep, an abundance of work you love, an abundance of time with your family.

In the scarcity culture we live in, I know this is easier said than done. Go against that culture. You are not your milk production. You are so much more than a milk-maker or a freezer stash.

CHAPTER 11

HALF A YEAR OLD, THEN SUDDENLY A BIRTHDAY (MONTHS SIX TO TWELVE)

MONTHS 6–9

FOR BREAST-FED BABIES: 5–8 feeds per 24 hours, but at more regular intervals

FOR BOTTLE-FED BABIES: 5–8 bottles of 4–6 ounces

Feedings become clustered into the day if a baby is weaned at night, adding complementary foods for extra calories and protein. Drinking water, formula, or breast milk from a cup as a bonus drink.

MONTHS 9–12

FOR BREAST-FED BABIES: 2–5 feeds, plus comfort nursing and snacking

FOR BOTTLE-FED BABIES: 2–5 bottles, 4–6 ounces

At this time, food transitions into being a meaningful part of a baby's diet, and they should use a cup for drinks. Milk becomes more of a supplement, and food becomes the core of their diet.

Welcome to the second half of the baby year! The second half of the baby year is all about exploring. In these next six months, your baby will explore your house, and every single thing they can put in their mouth. They will start sitting, then crawling, then walking. This can feel chaotic and overwhelming, since babies learn movement before they learn consequences. Try to find the fun in it wherever you can. Share foods you like and have experiences you can share. This is the iconic stuff of babyhood: exhausting, terrifying, and oh so rich.

You'll notice that these chapters are covering bigger chunks of time. That's because you are getting the hang of everything. Your knowledge of your kid and family is taking the reins. Things are less intense and new, but the six-month mark brings a big one: starting solid food. I encourage you to take a big loving look at your family foodways. Yes, the congee, the empanadas, the Chef Boyardee, the Renaissance fair turkey leg. Oral motor development follows gross motor development. As a baby has the core strength to sit up, they can also intentionally move their tongue to the side. The bilateral movement of crawling is associated with chewing and being able to chew foods. Follow your baby's lead developmentally as you start adding solids to their diet.

READINESS TO START SOLIDS

I was driving down the road listening to NPR when a story came on about Lucy's baby: the oldest baby specimen of humans. The hosts waxed poetically about how remarkable it was that her dental records indicated that she, like modern babies, started eating solid food around six months of age. This was a big ol' "yeah, duh" for me. If you have ever been around a baby who is ready for solids and is in the neighborhood of six months old, you know that they will straight up steal your sandwich. You can barely keep an interested baby away from solid food. Unless your doctor gives you a specific recommendation to start sooner, I encourage you to wait to start solids until your baby shows you they are ready by sitting independently. If your baby is ready to sit at the table, they are ready to start eating family meals.

A NOTE ABOUT ALLERGIES

If possible, reflect on your baby's genetics. If there are no signs of allergy in your baby in their genetic family, you can proceed with a wide variety of foods and only worry about allergies if there is a problem. If there are allergies in your family, you'll want to talk to a pediatric allergist for the most up-to-date information about when to introduce foods for the best chance at reducing allergic reactions long-term.

BABY-FOOD MAKERS

It's really easy to heat up frozen vegetables and mash them with a fork. A dedicated device is really unnecessary. If you like gadgets, then get an immersion blender. It's more versatile and will last longer into your life. They fit perfectly in mason jars for blending up whatever table foods you are sharing with your baby.

INTRODUCING SOLID FOOD

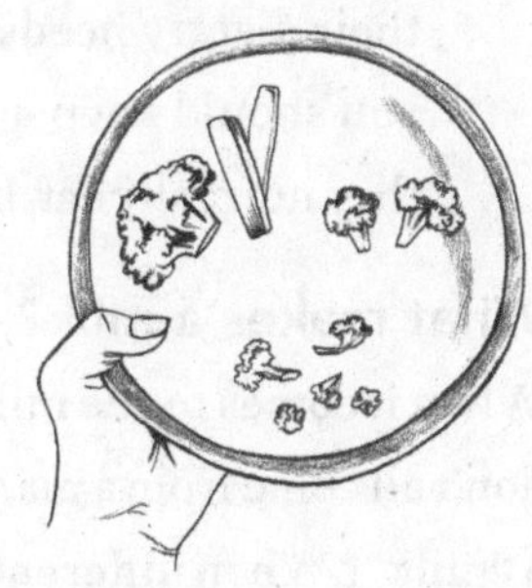

How to get started:

1. Focus on family foods, especially fruits and vegetables, and high-iron foods. Go to the grocery store and pick out some foods your family loves and have fun introducing them.
2. Use a variety of feeding methods. You'll find a lot of theories on how to offer foods to babies. In reality, different methods teach different skills. Start with a combination of purees or mashed table food on spoons, as well as some pieces for your baby to pick up. When offering pieces of food (often called "baby-led weaning"), start with larger chunks and gradually go smaller. This way your baby will gnaw on a larger piece while they work on chewing.
3. Start offering cups. Offering a cup of formula or expressed milk with meals as early as six months is a great start. Sippy cups teach kids to bite while they drink, which can also mess with teeth and speech. Start by holding the cup for your baby and very gradually tipping a little bit of the contents into their mouth and letting them work on swallowing. Eventually, they will want to hold the cup themselves and make their own messy attempts.

   For straw drinking, start by drawing some milk into a straw and capping it with your finger (like you would do with soda when you were eleven). Then, release a few drops at a time into your baby's mouth. Offer straw cups for exploring at mealtimes and give a lot of time and space to explore developing this new sucking technique.

4. Continue to offer bottles or nursing as a fundamental calorie source until one year old. At one year, most pediatricians feel good about babies moving on to having cow's milk or water with their meals. You may also nurse or do bottles beyond the magic one-year mark. All of that is family preference. What we know is that babies don't usually eat enough solid foods or drink well enough from cups to meet all of their dietary needs at the table until around their first birthday. So, you should keep adding solid foods and cup drinking above what they normally eat, but should not start cutting back until after a year.

What makes a milk?

When it comes to the milk we have at the grocery store, you'll notice they don't all come from a mammal. So why is rice drink a "drink" and pea milk a "milk"? When different milk alternatives started to come onto the market, the FDA classified them based on nutrition. In order to be classified as milk, a beverage has to have a certain amount of protein. Rice drink doesn't meet this cut-off and thus got reclassified. Also be mindful of flavorings. Flavored milks can be very high in sugar. I'm a big fan of allowing kids some sugar and being generally neutral about foods, but getting a lot of their calories from sugary beverages makes kids more likely to miss out on other foods and nutrients.

HOW TO FEED A TEETHING BABY

Teething lasts forever. When your baby is born, they have already made all of their teeth, and the way they emerge from the gums is still somewhat of a mystery. What we know is that babies "cut teeth" from the age of four months until about three years. They also have a wide range of experiences of cutting teeth. Some babies don't seem to notice, others have low fevers, excessive drooling, and disrupted sleep. Teething can also temporarily change feeding patterns. In a good suckle, babies use their tongue and lips to do all the work, and their teeth shouldn't be part of the equation. Some babies are comforted while teething by biting down on things, which can sometimes be a nipple: bottle or human. Sucking is powerful pain relief for babies, so they may also want to eat more often. Disrupted sleep can also lead to more sucking for comfort. If you are nursing and feel overtaxed, you can absolutely offer a bottle, pacifier, or teether.

If you are nursing and your baby is chomping while teething, you should use a fishhook finger (page 103) as a bite block and unlatch. Don't make a big deal about it, as that can reinforce the action. Just move on to your next activity and try nursing again later.

Teeth brushing

Once your baby has teeth, you need to brush them. If you are bottle feeding, you should brush them after their last bottle of the night. When we bottle feed, milk pools in the mouth and touches the teeth. When nursing, the way that the breast tissue fills the mouth means that milk doesn't pool in the same way. For this reason, with nursing, you should brush your baby's teeth in the evening, but you don't need to worry about it happening after the last feeding. Instead, brush teeth in the evening and morning as part of your bedtime and getting-ready routines.

WEANING

YOUR BODY DURING WEANING

There is frustratingly little research about what bodies go through during *involution*. This is the name for what our bodies go through during weaning off nursing or pumping. Many people report a significant hormonal change that feels similar to how they felt postpartum. For this reason, I recommend going slow. Going slowly can also reduce the chance of mastitis or other complications. If you are pumping, start by reducing your pumping volume by about a fourth every two days. For example, if you had been pumping four ounces, stop when you hit three. You can use the massage techniques on page 164 to stay comfortable. For nursings, it is easier to drop them one by one. If you are doing both, drop the pumping first. Then gradually drop out feedings. Start by dropping every other feeding. So, if you feed at 9:00, 12:00, and 3:00, for instance, start by dropping the 12:00 feeding and wait until your body feels comfortable between the 9:00 and 3:00 to drop another. You may find that even after you are completely done pumping or nursing your body still makes milk. This is very common. Once your body has turned on its milk-making system, it never fully turns it off again. It is sort of like a sleep mode on your computer. Your body no longer uses energy to make milk, but it stays in a more ready state to jump back in if called to action. This is why milk transitions more quickly with subsequent kids and it is easier to re-lactate if you decide you want to unwean.

If you are done before one year, you will replace nursing with bottles of formula to round out your baby's nutrition. Offer a bottle in place of a nursing session and gradually (over two weeks or so) work your way to all bottles. Going slowly will give your body time to adjust.

YEAR ONE AND BEYOND

FOR BREAST-FED BABIES: Nursing moves to a role of comforting and filling gaps in nutrition and immunology. This is sometimes 6,000 very short feedings or at wake-up or bedtime.

FOR BOTTLE-FED BABIES: Your baby no longer needs bottles and should be getting all of their nutrition from food and cups. Many families still offer bottles as comfort or habit. Talk to your child's dentist and pediatrician; if they think it's fine, I think it's fine.

Your baby's first birthday! This is a huge milestone for you.

Your baby now no longer needs breast milk or formula to get enough calories and nutrition, and can switch to drinking cow's milk or water. However, it is common to still nurse at beyond a year. This may be through the day and night, or just at wake-up and bedtime.

BREAST MILK AFTER A YEAR

After a nursling is a year old, milk transitions to being higher calorie to fill in nutritional gaps, while meeting their busy, frenzied nursing style. This means that even if your toddler nurses infrequently, they are getting extra calories to fill in their diet even with small volumes. Biologically, human milk, pumped or nursed, still represents part of a baby's immune system. The antibodies in a parent's milk still protect a child between one and three years old. Just like at any point in nursing, a theoretical health benefit doesn't mean you need to offer your milk. If you receive cultural pushback around doing so, this can be a helpful morsel of information to share.

At one year, how much milk does a baby need?

Your production is so stable at this point that you should be able to go long chunks without losing production. Very intermittent toddler nursing will not create the robust supply they had and needed when they were three or four months old, but it's the perfect volume for this age.

If you need to be away from your toddler but want to maintain some milk production for your return, try pumping with an electric or hand pump two to four times in twenty-four hours for five or ten minutes to still send the signal that milk is desired.

As toddlers venture into the world and develop into exploring more, they will often do what is called "rupture and repair." A toddler will venture away from you and reach the edge of where they are comfortable and miss you and come back, or maybe fall over and bump their head. When they come back, or you go to them, they often want a reassurance of your attachment. This can be a cuddle, some kind words, or nursing. Some people find it to be a cranky-toddler-soothing superpower.

Similarly, some kiddos who are in someone else's care during the day might do well by reconnecting at the end of the day with nursing. This is, as always with nursing, optional. If it feels right to you, stick with it. If it doesn't, then don't.

In many countries there is a stigma about nursing after age one. I find it obnoxious, but with all stigmas, you get to decide if you would like to subvert it or be private. Because of this, it's pretty common to only nurse toddlers at home before sleep or after waking. You probably know many more people who nursed their toddlers than you would think. How you want to be in public is your choice. I want to offer you a variety of options.

You can choose to *not* nurse your toddler, do so privately, or do so publicly. All are normal and good in my view.

And remember that in relationships you get to say yes and no, and you are teaching your child important skills around boundaries when you do this.

Toddler formulas

There are many toddler formulas on the market. Some of them are nutritionally very similar to infant formula but have not/do not want to jump through the hoops to pass the scrutiny to be labeled an infant formula. Some are very different from infant formula and resemble a meal-replacement shake. These tend to be pretty expensive when compared to food or plain cow's milk. Unless your pediatrician is concerned about your toddler's growth and suggests this, I say skip it. Instead, offer a smoothie or other table foods. At this point, milk should be consumed more as a drink than a meal replacement.

Weaning from bottles

It can be hard to let go of our little babies as they get older, but after the first birthday is a good time to start weaning from bottles. The suck pattern of bottles can impact teeth and speech development, so it is good to move to a straw cup or open cup instead. If bottles are associated with sleep for your child, start by eliminating them at all other times of the day and removing the bedtime and nap time bottles last. After you have moved the milk drinking into a cup, you can gradually move to where milk is positioned as a drink with meals, rather than a snack or meal itself.

It is very normal for kids to still want a lot of oral sensory input. Try offering a "chewy" for your kid to have at comforting times instead of a bottle. These can be attached to a necklace and come in all shapes and sizes.

At this point, the expectation is that your kid gets most of their calories from eating table foods and is supplementing their diet with human milk, formula, or cow's milk. These milks are all engineered by either modern food science or our bodies to give our kids the extra calories and vitamins they need. If you are still nursing and/or giving water but not offering formula or cow's milk, you should continue to offer vitamin D.

Weaning a toddler

If you wean after a year, there is no need to replace nursings with bottles. Most parents choose to start with the feedings in the middle of the day and work from there. The nursings first thing in the morning and before bed are usually the last to go. It is good to have conversations about what is happening, especially if your child is over two, explaining that you are all done nursing and that you are going to gradually stop. Offer alternatives, for example, another caregiver might need to do bedtime or wake-up to ease frustration around these times.

GETTING PREGNANT AGAIN

If you are trying to get pregnant again, you may find that nursing or pumping impacts your fertility. This is because prolactin can impact your ovulation. If getting pregnant is taking longer than you would like it to, you may want to talk to your OB-GYN, midwife, or reproductive endocrinologist (RE) about whether weaning might help.

Some people get pregnant easily or accidentally while nursing. Despite breastfeeding's impact on ovulation, it's pretty faulty as birth control. If you do not want another pregnancy, I highly recommend using another method of birth control.

Most people experience a drop in milk production and pain/discomfort with nursing once pregnant. This is due to the change in hormones starting the lactation process over again. This usually resolves in the second trimester. You can wean, or nurse through it. Some people nurse through their pregnancy and after the new baby is born. In late pregnancy, nursing is not a risk for preterm labor unless you have other risk factors or on pelvic rest. The rule here is "If you are allowed to have sex, you are allowed to nurse." The logic being that oxytocin, the hormone of letdown, orgasm, and contraction, is treated similarly regardless of how it is triggered.

TANDEM NURSING

Tandem nursing is when you nurse a new baby and older child at the same time. It's recommended that you nurse your new baby first, then your older child. This ensures that your little baby, who is more dependent on these calories, gets their fill before their sibling. For those that it is a good fit for, tandem nursing is an awesome experience. The toddler often has an easier time transitioning to having a new sibling, helps increase milk supply, and can help with clogs or engorgement.

Here we are, at the end. The end of your nursing or bottle-feeding road. For some of us, this is a huge relief; for others it comes with a lot of sadness. We all have different preferred phases of parenting. If you are all about that little baby phase, the leaving behind of baby-feeding tools can feel like the end of an era. Whereas some of you, I'm sure, can't wait to get to some of the more active and interactive seasons of parenting. I have nothing for you on picky eaters besides: They usually grow out of it. For eating with children in restaurants, all I can say is, "Tip well."

I hope that whatever you have left behind and whatever you are moving toward, this book has made you feel more confident and made you feel like enough, because you did it, you fed your baby! Maybe you fed multiple babies. I am so proud of you. I hope that beyond feeding your baby, you found some joy, and I hope you are proud of yourself.

SECTION FOUR

HELP FOR WHEN IT'S NOT WORKING.

CHAPTER 12

POSTPARTUM MOOD AND DEPRESSION

Let's talk a bit about mood. The combination of sleep deprivation, stress, and hormones happening after someone has a baby is a natural hotbed for what we call *postpartum mood disorders*. This includes depression and anxiety, but can also be obsessive-compulsive disorder (OCD), intrusive thoughts, insomnia, and in rare cases, hallucination and psychosis.

Co-parents can also have postpartum mood disorders. While the hormonal pathways of perinatal mood disorders are absolutely part of the picture, all parents can have perinatal mood disorders and are worthy of help. These can be driven by trauma during birth or postpartum or by sleep deprivation. This is all complicated by the lack of support out there on the subject, and for some people, a lot of gender performance to be a strong dad or parent and to support the family.

When I talk about feeding, I always talk about mood. Mental health can be enhanced by or devastated by feeding outcomes. It should also be a big part of how we make risk-benefit decisions about feeding our babies. If nursing is going well and supports your mood, that should be part of the equation.[19] If bottle feeding allows you to sleep enough to not need psychiatric intervention, that should be part of the assessment. If you need medication to help with mood or focus, you should take it knowing that some meds will be compatible with feeding your own milk (most of them) and some will not.

If you're struggling with mood at this or any point, refer to this checklist to help figure out where you're at.

POSTPARTUM MOOD AND DEPRESSION

STEP 1: SLEEP

Sleep is the top priority in families where anyone is struggling with mood. Try to stagger sleep with other caregivers so that you can get a chunk of four to six hours of protected sleep. Protected sleep means that you are assured that no one will need you during this time. Sleep as far from the rest of the family as possible, use white noise, earplugs, medication, melatonin, a warm bath. Whatever will help you sleep.

STEP 2: CHECK IN WITH YOURSELF

If you don't feel better after you've slept, or can't sleep when given the opportunity, it is time to seek help. Gender and stigma can make this hard, but caring for your mental health will make you a better caregiver, provider, partner, and parent. This is not lip service. Mood disorders do not go away on their own; they tend to get worse with time, which will eventually impact your family. So, take a moment to look at the big picture and see if you can identify what you need.

STEP 3: ACCESSING HELP

Talk to your partner, friends or primary care provider (PCP). If you don't have a PCP, you can actually talk to your birthing team. Even if you aren't a birthing parent, they will be able to connect you to resources. You should also talk to them about ways to aid in your sleep. They will not be able to prescribe medication for partners, but they can offer over-the-counter options where appropriate or refer you to someone who can prescribe.

If you are having dangerous intrusive thoughts or feel like you are a risk for harming yourself: Go to the ER. They are well-trained in helping stabilize people who are in mental health crisis. This can feel like a very scary step, with ideas of involuntary holds, but in reality, if you voluntarily seek help, you will be able to voluntarily leave once you've made a plan for follow-up with the hospital mental health team.

There is no "should" when it comes to how you feel, and chances are you will feel different from one day to the next (or even hour to hour). It's important to check in with yourself regularly. For this, meet the EPDS, or as I think of it, the very well-substantiated *Cosmo* quiz of mood disorders. This thing is tried and true and should be used early and often to check in on how you are doing. As someone who had severe postpartum mood disorders, I have taken this test *a lot*. I find it extremely annoying and you might also. It is, however, a really good tool so use it anyway.

No one will see this but you, unless you choose to show your doctor. Try not to be swayed by the point values as you take it and be as honest as you can.

EDINBURGH POSTNATAL DEPRESSION SCALE[20] (EPDS)

As you are pregnant or have recently had a baby, we would like to know how you are feeling.

Please check the answer that comes closest to how you have felt IN THE PAST 7 DAYS, not just how you feel today.

I have felt happy:

- ☐ **Yes, all the time (0)**
- ☐ **Yes, most of the time (1)**
- ☐ **No, not very often (2)**
- ☐ **No, not at all (3)**

This would mean: "I have felt happy most of the time" during the past week. Please complete the other questions in the same way.

In the past 7 days:

1. **I have been able to laugh and see the funny side of things**
   - ☐ **As much as I always could (0)**
   - ☐ **Not quite so much now (1)**
   - ☐ **Definitely not so much now (2)**
   - ☐ **Not at all (3)**

2. **I have looked forward with enjoyment to things**
   - ☐ **As much as I ever did (0)**
   - ☐ **Rather less than I used to (1)**

☐ Definitely less than I used to (2)

☐ Hardly at all (3)

3. I have blamed myself unnecessarily when things went wrong

☐ Yes, most of the time (3)

☐ Yes, some of the time (2)

☐ Not very often (1)

☐ No, never (0)

4. I have been anxious or worried for no good reason

☐ No, not at all (0)

☐ Hardly ever (1)

☐ Yes, sometimes (2)

☐ Yes, very often (3)

5. I have felt scared or panicky for no very good reason

☐ Yes, quite a lot (3)

☐ Yes, sometimes (2)

☐ No, not much (1)

☐ No, not at all (0)

6. Things have been getting on top of me

☐ Yes, most of the time I haven't been able to cope at all (3)

☐ Yes, sometimes I haven't been coping as well as usual (2)

☐ No, most of the time I have coped quite well (1)

☐ No, I have been coping as well as ever (0)

7. I have been so unhappy that I have had difficulty sleeping

☐ Yes, most of the time (3)

☐ Yes, sometimes (2)

☐ Not very often (1)

☐ No, not at all (0)

8. I have felt sad or miserable

☐ Yes, most of the time (3)

☐ Yes, quite often (2)

- ☐ **Not very often (1)**
- ☐ **No, not at all (0)**

9. I have been so unhappy that I have been crying

- ☐ **Yes, most of the time (3)**
- ☐ **Yes, quite often (2)**
- ☐ **Only occasionally (1)**
- ☐ **No, never (0)**

10. The thought of harming myself has occurred to me

- ☐ **Yes, quite often (3)**
- ☐ **Sometimes (2)**
- ☐ **Hardly ever (1)**
- ☐ **Never (0)**

If you scored:

10+: Tell someone and get help right away.

You are going to need more sleep, some meds, and support, but you aren't alone, you can feel better, and you deserve to feel better.

6–10: It's time to engage support.

Ask two friends or family members to make concrete plans to come spend time with you and help out. Plan at least one four- to six-hour chunk of protected sleep and a few naps, so that your sleep total is eight-plus hours in twenty-four hours. Call your PCP, midwife, or OB-GYN, and let them know that you aren't in an emergency, but you'd like to follow up. Call your therapist to check in if you have one.

6 or lower: You are in okay shape.

Having a new baby is hard, but your mood seems to be holding steady. Keep doing what you're doing.

Postpartum mood complications are the most common complication from giving birth. You are so far from alone. Here are some common ways people feel after having a baby.

"I don't feel connected to my baby"

This kind of disconnection or bonding is so normal. In the movies, after all manner of complex traumatic births, people hold their babies in their arms and everything is fine. In reality, it can be really hard to bond with a strange alien worm-looking thing. Especially if you have suffered trauma, are in pain, or that tiny creature cries all the time. Some people just really don't like the baby stage. All of these feelings are normal, and if you talk to someone about them, they just might reveal that they felt the same way. I know I did.

"I hate the way nursing makes me feel"

Nursing can feel weird. It can be too much touch or sensory input. It can trigger past trauma. It can just not feel right. Remember, store-bought is fine. If nursing doesn't feel right to you, you can switch to formula. Some people find pumping more comfortable, and that can work well, too. It is your body, and you get to choose what to do with it.

"Nursing triggers trauma from a past sexual assault"

Survivors of sexual assault have higher rates of a lot of nursing complications, including mastitis. It is perfectly reasonable to reclaim power in your body autonomy as a survivor and choose to feed your baby another way and to take breaks from skin-to-skin or even baby holding. Ask for support. Partners can be captain of skin-to-skin. Other family members can do the majority of the holding. This doesn't make you less of a parent.

"What if I hurt my baby? Hurt myself? Abandon my family?"

These intrusive thoughts are the hardest mood complication to get treatment for. They are usually a sign of obsessive-compulsive disorder (OCD). People often associate this diagnosis with repetitive actions or excessive cleanliness; in reality, it is categorized by intrusive thoughts. These thoughts can make it hard to sleep, hard to bond, and hard to connect with your community.

They can also make it hard to get treatment because of a fear that if someone finds out that you are thinking about harming yourself or your baby, they will report you. In truth, this is a greater risk for some people than others. Marginalized parents have a greater chance that an uneducated provider will report them. Some families, like Indigenous families, already have a long history of family separations and the removal of their children.

> **You are not alone, there is help out there, you deserve to feel better.**

I recommend talking to a birthing provider about this (your midwife or OB-GYN), because they have training in mood disorders, and using the words "intrusive thoughts" and explaining those intrusive thoughts.

"I ruined my life"

The dramatic change to having a baby can be really overwhelming. It can feel like your life is forever changed for the worse and there is no way out. Try talking to your support network about giving yourself time to do things you enjoyed before having a baby. This can be spending time with an older child, your partner or time alone doing things you love. Get more help with your baby and use tools like formula to get more time to be autonomous.

"I can't bear this. I want to die/I would be happy to just disappear"

Suicidal mood disorders are terrifying. I know because I had one. If you are having these thoughts, you should call the twenty-four-hour line of your birth provider, and if they can't be reached, go to the ER. They will give you safe medications to get you stable so you can get treatment. I was lucky enough to have Klonopin, a panic rescue med that is compatible with nursing, on hand. These drugs are helpful, and you should access them if you need them.

MY STORY

How do I know you aren't alone? Because I am right here with you. As I've alluded to, I am the survivor of a suicidal postpartum mood disorder, traumatic birth, and complex PTSD.

Before I was a parent, I was a parenting expert. I taught parenting skills, built infant feeding skills, and, with the help of other amazing doulas, built a community.

What I did not yet know was how much I would need to draw on these resources. How much I would be forced to walk the walk of all the talking I had done in my career.

Then, my family had an extremely traumatic birth. I say my family rather than "I" because my daughter's birth changed all three of us neurologically forever. While I wouldn't change my daughter's disability for the world, my struggle with PTSD has been the hardest challenge of my life. During our three-week NICU stay, I drew on depths of strength I never knew before. A week or two into my life as a "NICU mom," it became clear to me that I was in real trouble. The level of disassociation I was reaching was pushing on the line of postpartum psychosis.

Here is where my own story still blows my mind. I was in the hospital with the premier perinatal mood center for the entire country, if not world. UNC Hospitals was home to what at the time was the only specific perinatal psychiatric unit to allow infants into the clinic. Much of the research being done on these disorders was housed one floor below the NICU I was in. The icons of the field were feet away from me. And yet. The NICU I stood in was flooded with chaplains and neonatal care teams, but not a single therapist. I called my midwife. I reported my symptoms to my baby's nurse. I stood crying at the scheduling desk for the world-class perinatal mood clinic. My favorite midwife checked in, and I reported that I was drowning and couldn't seem to get any help. She took me by the hand and walked with me from psychiatric front desk to psychiatric front desk, until she finally convinced someone to get me an appointment that week.

It should not be this hard.

My spouse and I were able to see a psychology nurse practitioner at the hospital for the duration of my daughter's stay and for a few months thereafter. She prescribed us both drugs and helped us manage our acute symptoms.

Months later, on my thirtieth birthday, those drugs saved my life. We had gone to the beach for my birthday, and I genuinely could not bear to be in my head any longer. The dose of maintenance meds I was on was barely cutting it, and in hard moments couldn't touch my suffering. I was fully panicked, trapped in my own mind, and considering jumping off the balcony. Luckily, I had packed the rescue meds that had been prescribed to me. I was able to get down to the car, find them, take them, and go to bed. After that, my team was able to continue to adjust my medication. I entered very intensive therapy to treat my PTSD, and things got better.

The drugs to manage my symptoms were all safe for breastfeeding. And if I'm being honest, I'm not sure what I would have chosen if they weren't. I was indoctrinated to the idea of exclusively feeding my daughter my milk for six months. I know for certain that the pumping was making my mental and physical health worse, and I kept doing it. So, I don't know if I would have been brave enough to choose a medication that would have forced me to stop.

What I do know is that I will never stop fighting to make this better and easier for you. I repeat: IT SHOULDN'T BE THIS HARD. We all have to be vocal about our needs around mental health in hopes that the resources continue to multiply. These disorders are treatable, and you deserve to feel better. You do not have to sacrifice yourself on the altar of parenthood. You get to use any tool that allows you to thrive as a person first and a parent second. I also hear a lot about "You can't be a good parent unless you are well," and I find that true and not true at the same time. Mostly, I don't care. You are a person outside of parenting, and you deserve to be okay even if it doesn't benefit your kid.

Treating your mood disorder may look like: therapy, postpartum doula care, using formula, having your house professionally cleaned, exercise, medication, or meditation.

I also want to say that you can have a postpartum mood disorder that isn't hormonally driven. The transition to parenting can be destabilizing or traumatic for nonbirth parents as well. Partners are even less resourced in perinatal mood disorders and they (you, if you're reading this) deserve to thrive, too. Adoptive parents and parents through surrogacy can also be forgotten in this conversation, and shouldn't be.

All parents can have perinatal mood disorders and are worthy of help. Some common ones are OCD, PTSD, depression, or anxiety. These can be driven by trauma during observing birth or postpartum or by sleep deprivation.

> Dads, you are the least likely to get specific mental health support postpartum. You can still be a strong dad or parent and to support your family while asking for help. Asking for help can be range from taking a walk with a friend who has kids to seeking out a counselor. You may want to talk to your doctor about your own hormone levels and see if medication might help. You deserve support too.

MAKING A FEEDING PLAN TO SUPPORT YOUR MOOD

It is okay to change your feeding plan to meet the needs of your mood. I desperately wish that I had been able to fully believe this. My whole family would have been better off if I had stopped pumping and started formula feeding sooner. Do better than me. Choose your family's wellbeing.

The number-one goal in treating a postpartum mood disorder is eight total hours of sleep per twenty-four hours, with at least four to six of those consolidated and uninterrupted.

If you are formula feeding, this is a matter of getting help for those hours so that someone else can be in charge of the baby and you can go have a larger consolidated rest.

If you are nursing, feed your baby before the time when you will have help to get protected sleep. This doesn't have to be at night, but you may need blackout curtains if it isn't. Nurse your baby, pump, and go to sleep. Let your care team use pacifiers, walks in carriers, and whatever food source works so that you know you won't be interrupted for four to six hours. Once you wake up, feed your baby, and resume however you were feeding. Remember, you will still need a few naps to get to the eight hours per twenty-four.

CHAPTER 13

SPECIAL CIRCUMSTANCES

Every year I visit my alma mater of UNC-Chapel Hill to give a lecture on "special circumstances." In that lecture, and here, I'll cover multiples, disaster preparedness, and loss. These are not at the back because they are secret or less important, but because they span the entire scope of this book and deserve dedicated attention.

FEEDING MULTIPLES

Finding out you are having multiples is a little bit of a shock to the system. The good news is that people understand this is hard and, barring a global pandemic, tend to show up for you. Utilize any and all help that is offered.

As your body prepares for multiples, the placental lactogen hormones tell your body: There is more than one kid in here, so get ready. Your body then actually creates more milk-making tissue in proportion to the amount of placenta in your body. That being said, bodies aren't perfect and depending on your risk factors, your production may be high, or it may be low. Generally speaking, people can produce enough milk for two babies; three or more is a stretch. I've known people to nurse triplets, but it is rare, both because of milk production and how much extra time it adds to the already major work of caring for three or more babies.

First, check in with yourself and your team: what is most important to you about feeding these babies? How comfortable are you using bottles or formula? Do you want to nurse at all? I love the examples of Dani (page 116) and Andy (page 87), who both fed multiples different ways. Dani desperately wanted to nurse her babies, but the barriers were just too great, so she formula fed and comfort nursed her daughters after bottle feedings. Andy's wife had planned to nurse both babies, but upon realizing that they would need to divide and conquer, Arley exclusively formula fed one baby while his wife exclusively nursed the other.

Try to remember, babies are individuals, and it is okay to treat them that way. Starting by getting to know your multiples as individuals will serve you their whole lives.

You are also more likely to experience some amount of time in the NICU with multiples. Many twins skip the NICU all together these days, but I think it is helpful to wrap your head around the NICU ahead of time.

While most babies in the NICU eventually have the chance to work on nursing, they almost always need some pumped milk or formula, if only because adults can't sleep over in many NICUs—and honestly, it's high stress, and you need to get some sleep. So, if you want to provide your own milk for your baby, it is important to make a good pumping plan for the NICU. For example, will you be going back and forth from home? Do you want one pumping system at home and one at the hospital? Some people prefer to take their pumping supplies back and forth.

Personally, I preferred my personal hospital-grade pump over the one the NICU provided and only used theirs in a pinch. It is worth taking some time to think through these things and make a plan for the early days. I also recommend thinking about your pumping within a twenty-four-hour cycle. If you can comfortably do so, cluster your pumping in the daytime, and at night, pump before bed, once in the middle of the night, and again when you wake up.

What to pack if you anticipate a NICU stay:

- Your pump and supplies, if you would like to have your own
- Comfy layers of clothing that will allow you to pump but have privacy. (I pumped openly in front of many neurologists, who were, quite honestly, uncomfortable. This didn't bother me in the slightest, but watching specialists squirm may not be your hobby.)

- A soft cooler to take milk into the hospital
- A small container of dish soap
- Good socks with grips
- A truly enormous water bottle
- Valet passes
- A truly enormous Starbucks gift card

When your babies are born (or if they are too little to eat just yet, when they are ready for oral feeds), you will start by feeding one baby at a time. Multiples are even more squished than singletons and so they are even more likely to have side preferences or quirks to their nursing while they get oriented (page 57). I particularly recommend bodywork for all multiples to help with feeding and to prevent torticollis or helmeting.

Feeding one baby at a time allows you to figure out what side they nurse best on, how they eat most comfortably, who needs more time or support to latch.

If you are planning to nurse, for the first two weeks while you are getting the hang of things, my recipe to prioritize help/mental wellness and feeding options is this:

Goals: Nurse each baby at least 2 times per 24 hours. Express milk (by nursing or pumping on both sides) 6–12 times per 24 hours.

If you have help: Sleep while you have help and let helpers feed babies bottles of pumped milk or formula. Ideally you would get a 4- to 6-hour chunk of protected sleep every 24 hours.

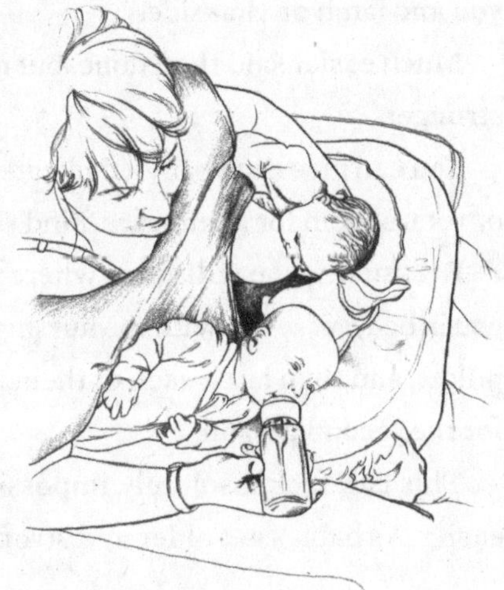

Some people have lots of help and find that pumping while others do bottles is easiest, while some people find that nursing two babies is the most efficient. It all depends on you, the help you have, and how your individual babies eat. You may find that one baby is a better nurser, or one really just prefers bottles. It is okay to feed different kids different ways.

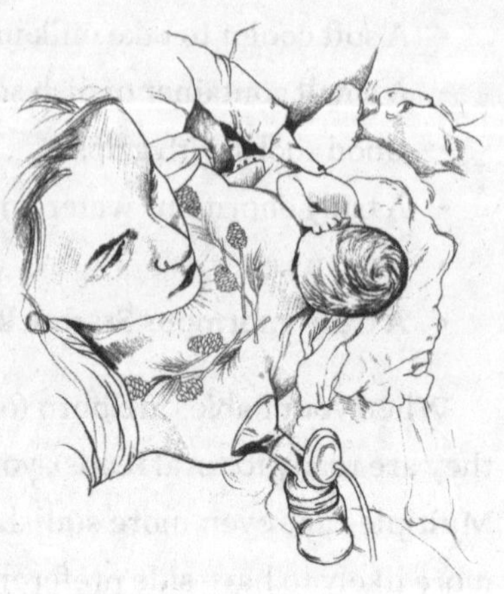

Supplies you'll need to nurse multiples:

- A truly enormous nursing pillow designed for twins, or a lot of bed pillows and towels.
- A second set of hands for the early days
- Rolled-up receiving blankets
- Possibly Kinesio Tape (page 131 for how this works)

Get all the way set up comfortably with your nursing surface and have one baby brought to you. Latch that baby and place a receiving blanket behind them for support. (If you figure out that your chest has to be held a certain way to maintain a comfortable latch, you can do this with Kinesio Tape to free up hands. K-Tape can stay on for several days and should be removed using oil.)

Once you have freed up your hands, have the second baby brought to you and latch on that side.

Much easier said than done, but it will get easier as they get bigger and stronger.

You can give each baby a dedicated side that they set the production on, or rotate them for symmetry. Find the way that works for you.

Eventually, you will get to where you can set the babies on either side of you in bed, get set up with the nursing pillow, put both babies on the nursing pillow, and then latch each of them from there, thus eliminating the need for the second person.

This can feel absolutely impossible in the early days, but it does get easier. As babies get older and stronger, they participate more and more in their own feeding. Eventually, putting in twice the work has twice the payoff when you can sit down and easily feed and soothe two babies at once.

BOTTLE FEEDING MULTIPLES

Pumping

Some parents find that the best way to utilize the help they have or offer their multiples their milk is to exclusively pump—especially after a NICU stay where parents get very used to and good at pumping. If this fits into your lifestyle, awesome, see page 153 on exclusive pumping to set yourself up for success.

Formula feeding

Your babies may come home as preterms and still need premixed sterile formula, this is the most expensive formula, but it just is what some babies need. You can ask your pediatrician or WIC office for samples and coupons and move on to mixing formula at home as soon as your medical team thinks it's safe.

If you are formula feeding multiples, a good bottle-prep routine will be very helpful and allow you or a helper to get you set up for the day ahead. I recommend skipping the formula-making machine, as you are unlikely to have the time to routinely clean it and the measurements on them have been faulty in the past. Formula is instant, so mixing it on the fly works great.

Mix a pitcher. Mix twenty-four hours' worth of formula for your babies in a pitcher in the fridge. To do this, you will fill a pitcher with the appropriate amount of water. Then, in a separate bowl, measure your scoops. The reason to do this in a separate bowl is because if you miscount, you can just start over. Once you have counted out your scoops, pour that bowl of formula powder into the pitcher and stir. You can then pour from this pitcher into bottles throughout the day. Many babies are happy to eat cold bottles, but you can also pop these bottles into a bottle warmer or warm mug of water if you have a temperature-picky baby—or babies.

Make twenty-four hours' worth of bottles. You can also premake each individual bottle. This is great if you have many caregivers coming and going. Formula should only stay in the fridge for twenty-four hours, so you would fill all of the bottles you need for the day with water and add scoops to them. You can then use Post-its to label when and/or who each bottle is for.

Mix as you go. If you are less of a meal prep person, set yourself up to make bottles as you go. I recommend either an electric kettle with a temperature readout or a pitcher of water that remains on the counter at room temperature. You can just add the water and formula powder to bottles as you go. If your baby is pre-term and you don't have well water, you can also use water right from the faucet, but be careful about temperatures: sometimes water is hotter than we realize.

SAFER PROPPED BOTTLES

In a perfect world, you would never have to prop a bottle and would have one dedicated, loving adult to do every feeding for every baby, every time. This is the safest and best way to do bottles, but we are not purists around here, and there will be times when you just don't have enough hands. So, rather than getting a bottle-holding device, try doing a side-lying bottle that is supported by a rolled blanket.

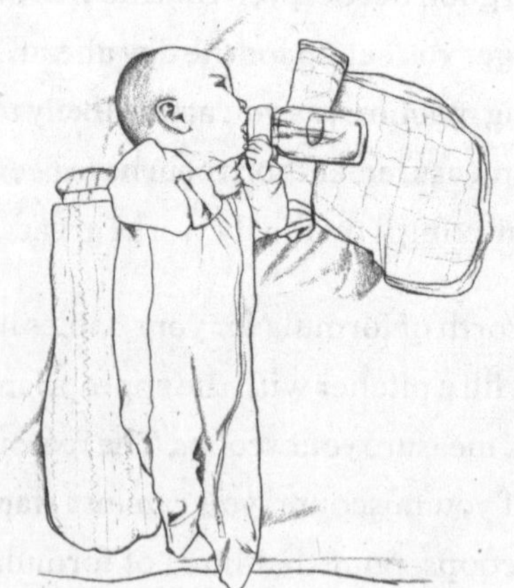

This is absolutely something you should do while supervising, but can also be done when there are more babies than caregivers around.

SPECIALIZED FEEDING TOOLS

SUPPLEMENTARY NURSING SYSTEM

A supplementary nursing system, or SNS, is a prosthetic system that allows people with low or no milk flow to chest feed. It is either a bottle or a milk necklace attached a thin tube that is taped along your chest to your nipple. This gives you and your baby the experience of nursing while using formula or donor milk for the calories. This may work great for you, but I find it quite finicky for those high-stress early days. It works better as a long-term supplement option. Adoptive nursers, trans nursers, people who have had surgery on their chests, or people with insufficient glandular tissue are all great SNS candidates. It can take some trial and error to get used to, but if nurturing at your chest/breast is important to you and you don't make milk or don't make enough milk, this is an excellent tool. If you make some milk, this also gives you the ability to get the stimulation of nursing while supplementing at the same time, which will help maintain or increase production.

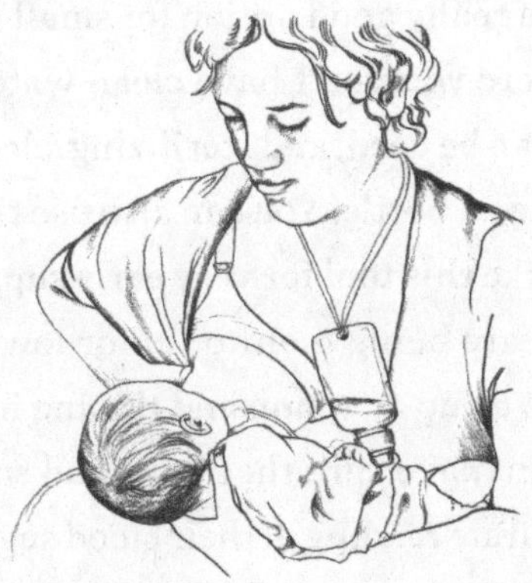

SYRINGE FEEDING

Syringe feeding is another way to avoid bottles with early supplementation. If I'm being honest: It's not my go-to tool. I think that if your baby needs

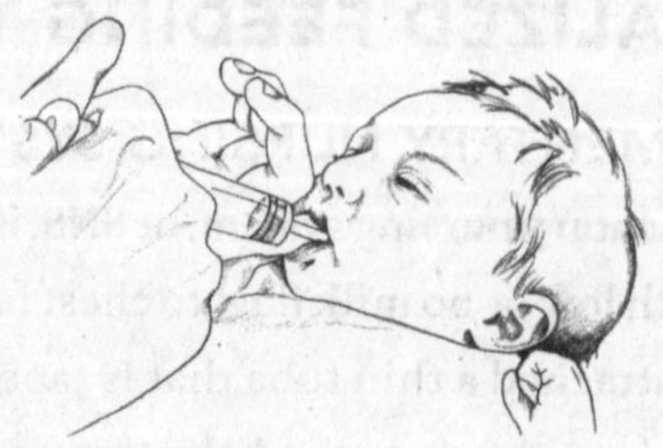

syringe feeding, they probably also need some suck training, which is better done by paced bottle feeding. If avoiding bottles altogether is important to you, however, this is an option. You draw milk up into a specialized syringe and slowly drip it into the corner of a baby's mouth while they nurse or suck on a finger. This option gives you a lot of control over flow, which enables you to incentivize good sucking skills.

CUP OR SPOON FEEDING

Cup feeding has been shown to decrease dependence on bottles and is a really good option for small volumes or in situations where you don't have clean water. Clean disposable cups can be used, and sterilizing/cleaning a cup is easier and takes less water than a bottle. You can also use this technique with a spoon. I particularly like this tool for very early supplementation of colostrum for babies who are being monitored for low blood sugar. By hand expressing milk into a cup or spoon and tipping it into a baby's mouth, you can make sure they have had some milk and get a more accurate reading of their blood sugar (page 185).

Simply tip the cup or spoon so milk pools at the edge and let your baby lap at it like a kitten.

HABERMAN BOTTLE

Babies with cleft palates and with some neurological conditions cannot suck. This can be because they can't make a vacuum or because they can't coordinate a suck. These bottles work on compression instead of suction. A one-way valve lets milk flow into the tip of the nipple and not back out into the bottle so a baby can bring it into their mouth by compressing the nipple. This is a specialized tool that will be given and taught to you by your medical team if you need it.

FEEDING TUBE

I love feeding tubes. I am the parent of a NICU graduate, and a feeding tube without a doubt saved her life and the lives of several of our friends. I was also terrified of feeding tubes in the early days. To me, they signified a difference or disability I wasn't ready to deal with yet. These tools are really common to use in preemies and other babies who are having trouble figuring out how to eat. They are also often used for babies who will need surgery and need to gain weight quickly or those who burn more calories than they can keep up with due to an underlying condition. Some people may use them their whole lives, and some people may need them for a short time. The beauty of a feeding tube is that they are removable. If you no longer need it, you remove it. The two primary feeding tubes for young babies are nasogastric tube (NG tube) and gastric feeding tube (G tube). An NG tube goes down the nose and throat to the stomach. A pump or syringe is connected to the tube and pushes milk or formula into the tube to feed a baby. They can make sucking harder because of the sensation at the back of the throat. They also give us a great feeding option without surgery.

A G tube (or J tube or any other feeding tube that goes directly to lower digestion) is placed during a routine surgery. Surgery never feels minor on our baby and puts some kids at risk of other complications. It can also feel scary and permanent. It is not. A G tube is like an extreme belly piercing and can be removed at any time without surgery and left to heal. In fact, they heal so quickly that if a G tube comes out, you need to replace it in a matter of hours before it starts healing closed. They can also be left in to be used as needed. If your baby starts eating primarily by mouth, you can keep the G port for medication or for fluids and food when your baby is sick.

People with feeding tubes can still eat by mouth. This gives many families the chance to work on feeding and sucking skills without stressing about calories and volumes. It allows families the chance to go about their lives and not spend every moment feeding.

Feeding tubes are a tool, and I encourage you to never fear a tool. I know how much easier said than done this is, but I promise: tubies are awesome.

MILK PRODUCTION AFTER LOSS

Pregnancy and infant loss are hard to talk about. Most people want to ignore them all together, but this book is about inclusion and honesty, and loss is part of reproduction. If you are not in a place to engage with loss, go ahead and skip this section. If you have experienced a loss, know that you and your babies are welcome here, even when others shy away.

If you experience the loss of a pregnancy or baby after about 16 weeks' gestation, you may experience a milk transition or produce milk after your baby is gone. People experience this differently. For some, immediately stopping milk production (known as "drying off") is important, and for others, producing milk in honor of their baby is a healing experience. Whatever supports your grief is right. You should know that if conceiving again soon after your loss is a goal, lactation can delay the process of your body returning to a state where you can get pregnant.

DRYING OFF

You can talk to your doctor about using medication or herbal remedies to stop milk production. You can also use the lymphatic drainage techniques to stay comfortable while leaving your chest full. Over the course of a few weeks your production will stop; sooner, if aided by medication.

EXPRESSING AFTER LOSS

If you want to produce milk for donation to other babies, either through peer donation or a milk bank, you can continue lactating by expressing

ALLIE AND DEXTER'S STORY

After Dexter died, the midwives asked what I wanted to do about my milk. They knew I had hoped to breastfeed. They told me that there were systems in place to support donating milk, but that I didn't have to pursue that if I didn't want to. Milk donation sounded helpful to me; it sounded like something I could focus my attention on instead of missing the baby I desperately wanted to hold. The midwives gave me a few suggestions, and I started pumping while I figured out what I would do next.

I didn't want to do more bloodwork, answer more questions about the raw wounds of infant loss, explain to yet another hospital system and team of providers that my baby was dead and it wasn't my fault. I wasn't even sure yet that it wasn't my fault. So, instead of donating to a milk bank, peer donation felt right for me.

I posted to the new parent group from our birth doulas and several moms connected me directly to families looking for breast milk. Pumping was a productive action that helped my grief, and I felt that it also helped my body heal, my uterus shrink, my still-seemingly-pregnant body disappear back into a nonpregnant state. My lactating body kept producing milk for whomever could use it next.

I donated to two families, one who moved across the country with their trunk full of my milk stash, and the other with a daughter who was born three days after my son. It was an instant overlap I hadn't realized I needed. They came to our home with their beautiful baby, listened to our story, and cried with us while I held her. She was the first infant I held after my son died. Our relationship evolved; we shared meals and stories, talked about the complexities of growing our families. They kindly offered to let me nurse their daughter, something I couldn't bring myself to do, and I will never forget how much more like a mama that offer made me feel. Their daughter has grown into a funny, strong, beloved human, and it bittersweetly warms my heart to see her reach the milestones my first son will never have. As I weaned, dropping pumping sessions slowly over time, I cherished every interaction we had and learned a lot from our shared vulnerabilities.

(continues)

This family shared many joyful events with us, including sharing excitement and then tears over our next pregnancy, briefly lived before an early miscarriage.

My third pregnancy was uneventful aside from the global COVID-19 pandemic that closed hospitals to doulas, photographers, and visitors ten days before my partner and I experienced the birth of our living son.

The light switch of change that occurs once the breathing, moving tiny human you created lands on your chest is indescribable. Transitioning to breastfeeding was both foreign and natural, as my body dutifully did everything I asked of it. I fought to learn, to get my questions answered, and to combine IBCLC guidance with what I was capable of handling through the challenges of postpartum hormonal changes complicated by both bliss and grief. The grief never goes away.

As my son aged and grew in strength we added solids, we taught him how to use a variety of cups, we watched him explore food. While he excitedly tried new foods, he continued to breastfeed eagerly for months . . . until one day he didn't. He was a little over fourteen months when he weaned himself. I cried, I questioned myself, I worried about the many things I'd done wrong to lead to this point. I wondered how I couldn't have realized the last latched feed was truly the last; I would have cherished it more! My spouse tried hard to reassure me: I had given my son so much milk with my body for so long, and this was simply another chapter.

For us, the next transition was to exclusive pumping, as if I had come full circle with my living child. I pumped four or five times a day to produce enough milk, and my son happily guzzled human milk from his favorite cups.

As I write, we are almost twenty-one months into my son's human milk consumption, and I'm trying to make it until he turns two.

The only reliable thing in this human growing experience is change, and while I'm not sure I'm ready for what's next, I know we'll figure it out.

milk. Pump or hand express if you feel uncomfortably full or at times of day when you feel like you need to. Your production will adjust to whatever schedule feels right, and any family that receives this milk will be grateful for it and will have been helped by you and your child.

DISASTER PREPAREDNESS

Unfortunately, natural disasters are getting more and more common. In my time as a lactation consultant, I've known parents to have to evacuate due to fire or flood, and be separated from their babies by washed out bridges. I've seen the most resourced families on the planet bring newborns home to no heat, no power, no clean water, and subfreezing temperatures.

Nothing can truly prepare you for disaster, but speaking as someone who grew up in earthquake country, we can at least have supplies on hand.

Always have some water and formula on hand—even if you are exclusively nursing. This is a great thing to do with samples that are mailed to you during your pregnancy. Even if it isn't your preferred brand or style of formula, it will do in a disaster.

Keep either individual bottles of shelf-stable formula—the advantage of the individual bottles is that you can keep disposable nipples on hand and just screw them on—or packets/cans of dried formula and enough bottled water for seventy-two hours of feeding and washing bottles. Keep at least three bottles with your emergency kit, along with some sanitizing wipes.

If your baby has significant food allergies, then you will need to have hypoallergenic formula on hand.

If you are nursing, keep an extra hand pump and disinfecting wipes with your emergency supplies. I strongly recommend practicing hand expression skills to stay comfortable and mastitis-free if you are separated from your baby. If you are a full prepper, you can keep a cooler and crackable ice packs in your kit to keep your stash cold during an evacuation.

If you lose power due to snow and ice, you can remove your freezer stash and put it outside, where temperatures may stay colder than inside your fridge and freezer.

FORMULA SHORTAGE AND CONTAMINATION

During the writing of this book, my perspective on disaster preparedness shifted again. When a major formula production plant was shut down, a formula drought hit the United States. While I feel strongly that this is not an individual issue and we need to work on a national and global level to prevent this kind of crisis, I do think it is something to be prepared for.

Firstly, recalls happen. While the ripple effect of this recall was much greater than others have been, it is a good idea to snap a photo of the lot number on the formula can you are using. This is the simplest way I have found to track this information in case of a recall—unless you are really into spreadsheets.

Keep two weeks' worth of formula in your pantry. This way you have a buffer to either transition gradually to another brand, share with a neighbor, or feed your baby while you wait for shelves to refill.

ᴧᴧᴧᴧᴧ

There is no way to prepare for and predict every circumstance; we can't live in fear of everything. My experience of the formula shortage was one of rage, yes, but also one of deep gratitude. Sharing saved us. Parents shared their beloved freezer stashes and extra formula. People mailed hypoallergenic options across the country to babies in need. We took care of each other, and that is a beautiful thing.

AFTERWORD

The hardest and best part of having kids is that they grow.

Time moves through us, and our babies need us a little less and a little less. There is a relief to this, and also a grief in this growing. For some parents, this goes lightning fast; for some of us, it happens steady and slow. Day by day we get further and further from when our babies needed us for everything. From feeding them every two hours to suddenly refusing to give them a snack too close to dinner.

You've also changed and grown through this process. You can't help it: parenting changes you no matter how you do it. Personally, I was laid bare by the first year of parenting. I melted like wax and reformed into the woman I am now. I've become more patient and more open to other people's realities. I know so much more about the sheer breadth of human experience. I'm definitely better medicated. My kid, now a preschooler, eats huge amounts of only a few foods, and I try not to get too in my head about it. We bake together with her standing in a learning tower and oats scatter across the floor as the measuring cup just misses the bowl. She eats chocolate chips right off the counter pressing her face right into the little pile. It is just as messy and frustrating as feeding her little infant self. It's also fleeting and beautiful and ours.

Infant feeding can feel like such a badge of individual identity, slowly fading into a family identity as your kid solidifies a new generation. Our families carry our food traditions. A through line that often outlasts us in the cycle of life. You'll make your child a dish your grandmother made, and somehow her legacy reaches through the generations right to your child.

After all the pressures of how to feed our babies, we feed our children. Just like infant feeding, it's imperfect and exhausting at times (dinner? Again? Really?), and it is enough.

That is my sincerest wish for you, just as it was all through this book: I hope you feel like enough. I hope you feel like the hard choices you made were enough. The nutrition you gave from your body or your kitchen shelf were enough. There is a reason we care so much about how we feed our babies: it is a real communion. We bond with them; we show our love through giving. We protect them by making the best choices we can, and if we are lucky, there is enough time and energy and love left over for ourselves. I'm finally feeling like enough for myself, my family and my kid. I hope you find yourself here, too. Even in the times of burnout and overwhelm: I hope you always come back to a homeostasis that even at your crummiest, you are still enough. Maybe when you don't feel it on your own, you can say to yourself: *Victoria thinks I'm enough*. Because I do.

APPENDIX

MILK STASH CALCULATOR

You may have heard people talking about their "milk stash." This is their bonus stock of milk that acts as a buffer for this renewable resource, to dip into when needed, like unexpected travel or surgery. When it comes to a stash, bigger isn't necessarily better. What I want you to think about is: How much milk do I need to have stored to feel secure? Just like with money, there are spenders and savers. You can put in the time filling deep freezers with milk, or you can pump today what your kid needs tomorrow. Either option can feel freeing or limiting to different people.

Let me be your lactation financial planner for a moment, and let's imagine some scenarios. Be as honest with yourself as you can.

- Your appendix burst (this is actually way common postpartum; weird, I know). With all the pain and hoopla and anaesthesia, you will not be able to feed your baby for the twenty-four hours that you are unexpectedly away. How much stress would be added to the situation by the idea of your baby getting formula during this time? Choose a number between 0 and 10, with 0 being "Who cares at a time like this?" and 10 being "That sounds worse than the appendicitis."

- You have been pumping at work and your supply has started to decrease now that your six-month-old baby BLESSEDLY sleeps through the night. Are you okay with gradually moving your baby to more solid food or adding formula to their routine? 0 being "Yeah, food after six months is fine, and formula is food," 10 being "That would feel like underperforming and really stresses me out."

- Your best friend is getting married last minute, a cute, simple courthouse thing. She wants you to come down for the weekend and celebrate with her. Your support system is more than happy to watch the baby, but you don't have enough milk stashed to cover the weekend. 0: "That's fine, I'll pump extra from now until then and make a plan"; 10: "That's too stressful. I'd rather skip the trip/bring the baby with me."

- You absentmindedly put your bag with your milk stash on the counter while digging into your ice cream stash at the back of the freezer. All of it thawed and you aren't going to be able to use it in the next 24–48 hours. How upset are you? 0: "It's fine, it's a renewable resource"; 10: "That was so. much. work. No one talk to me for at least a day."

Based on what you learned in that quiz, roughly outline your stash. If you got a low score, a small stash will work for you. If your score was high, you'll want to prioritize a bigger stash.

To feel secure, I would like to "stash" enough milk for (specify the number of hours you would like to have stash for):

__________ Outings

__________ Workdays

__________ Emergency away hours

Do you travel for work?

What is the longest you are likely to be away without your baby or a way to get milk home?

If you would like to leave breast milk for a trip, how many hours will you be away? __________

Other hours away that are currently planned: __________

About how many hours total (add up all the hours above)?

We roughly estimate that a baby eats one ounce per hour, so roughly approximate the number of hours you stated above, and that's how many ounces you will need to stash.

PRINTABLE FEEDING TRACKER

DAY 24 hour days from your baby's time of birth ____________

	1	2	3	4	5	6	7	8	9	10	11	12
Feedings	☐	☐	☐	☐	☐	☐	☐	☐	☐	☐	☐	☐
Bottle feeding (check box or fill with number of ounces)	☐	☐	☐	☐	☐	☐	☐	☐	☐	☐	☐	☐
Pumping/ expression	☐	☐	☐	☐	☐	☐	☐	☐	☐	☐	☐	☐
Chest was well drained (by feeding or expression)	☐	☐	☐	☐	☐	☐	☐	☐	☐	☐	☐	☐
Poops	☐	☐	☐	☐	☐	☐						
Pees	☐	☐	☐	☐	☐	☐						

Feeding Track any category that is helpful by rating that aspect of the feeding on a scae of 0 (low/bad)–10 (high/good)

Time started	Latch comfort	Quality of suck	Well drained/effective bottle eating	Feeding overall	Notes

BABY POOP TRANSITION CHART

Stooling Patterns of Exclusively Breastfed Babies

Time Period	# per Day	Appearance/Color	Amount
0–2 days	2–4	Meconium (black, thick tarry)	Scant to copious
3–4* days	2–5	Black to green to yellow, looser	Increasing volume
4–7 days	2–6+	Yellow, seedy, runny to loose	Copious by day 6 (4–8 stools/day)
1–6 weeks	3–8+	Yellow, seedy, runny to loose	Copious
6 weeks to 6 months	3–5+; may skip days	Yellow; soft; may thicken over time because of milk compositional changes	Copious, may be passed less often
6 months and onward		Loose; color and aroma may change as family foods are added	

*Fewer than 4 stools per day on or after day 4 should be investigated carefully.

MILK TRANSITION HORMONES

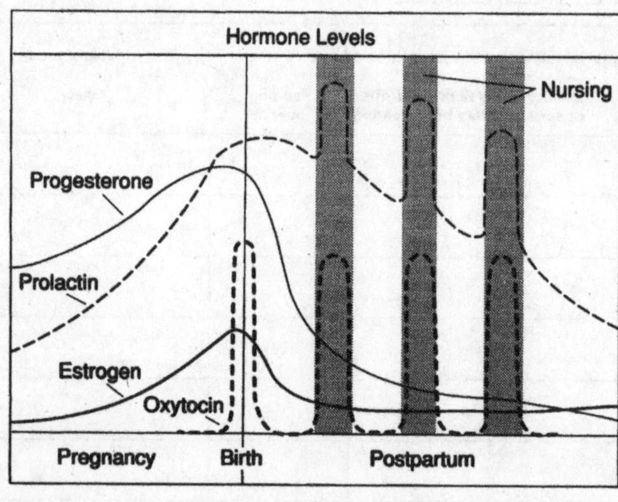

Karen Wambach and Jan Riordan, *Breastfeeding and Human Lactation, Fifth Edition*, 2009: Jones & Bartlett Learning, Burlington, MA. www.jblearning.com. Reprinted with permission.

ACKNOWLEDGMENTS

Getting to write a book is a privilege and an honor, so here I say thank you to everyone who participated in making my dream of getting these resources to families come true.

Thank you to Abby Olena and R Stein Wexler who got this book out of my mind and into the hands of my wonderful agent, Laura Usselman. Laura, thanks for always being there when I did the professional equivalent of yelling "MOM!" from the other room. To Maya Goldfarb, Jess Murphy, Rebecca Homiski, Rhina Garcia, Devorah Backman for helping me launch this very unwieldy project. I also thank Ann Treistman and Sam Eades for believing this book should exist and making it so. Helen Whitaker, Allison Chi, and Ashley Patrick; thank you for your brilliant minds. I am beyond lucky to have been helped along by so many brilliant women with complimentary skill sets.

To everyone who contributed a story or a photo to this book, thank you for making the book rich, vibrant and full of life. Thank you to Morgan and Arley for knowing everything I don't. Thank you to the Emerald Doulas for giving me my start.

Thank you to Ayden Love who made this book beautiful and being my partner in developing so many of the theories and ideas in this book. It is a joy to share so much overlap in love, friendship, work, and family. To Dr. Ellen Chetwynd and Dr. Maryanne Perrin, thank you for your mentorship and willingness to meet my endless questions with curiosity and collaboration.

Thank you, Anna, for making sure my kid was well loved and cared for while I wrote. Thank you to Melanie and Chaya, who keep my road from feeling lonely. To the Alpacas, who were my guinea pigs and are now my saving grace. To my queer family, who show up always. To the Jespersens, who are my port in a storm. To JulieAnna, who has listened to me pretend to be an expert since basically birth. To my dad, Julio, who gave me a deep love for all things peer reviewed and a shrewd skepticism of all absolutes.

And, mostly, to Jessie. Your love and encouragement is the greatest gift in my life, and I am so glad we spend too much time together.

NOTES

1. M. Vekemans, "Postpartum Contraception: The Lactational Amenorrhea Method," *The European Journal of Contraceptive Reproductive Health Care* 2, no. 2 (1997):105–11, doi: 10.3109/13625189709167463.
2. Juliette Herzhaft-Le Roy, Marianne Xhignesse, Isabelle Gaboury, "Efficacy of an Osteopathic Treatment Coupled with Lactation Consultations for Infants' Biomechanical Sucking Difficulties: A Randomized Controlled Trial," *Journal of Human Lactation* 33, no. 1 (2017): 165–72, doi: 10.1177/0890334416679620.
3. Michael S. Kramer, Beverley Chalmers, Ellen D. Hodnett, et al., "Promotion of Breastfeeding Intervention Trial (PROBIT): a randomized trial in the Republic of Belarus," *Journal of the American Medical Association* 285, no. 4 (2001): 413–20. doi: 10.1001/jama.285.4.413.
4. Maryanne T. Perrin, Roman Pawlak, Lisa L. Dean, Amber Christis, and Linda Friend, "A Cross-Sectional Study of Fatty Acids and Brain-Derived Neurotrophic Factor (BDNF) in Human Milk from Lactating Women Following Vegan, Vegetarian, and Omnivore Diets," *European Journal of Nutrition* 58, no. 6 (2019): 2401–10. doi: 10.1007/s00394-018-1793-z.
5. "Alcohol," *Drugs and Lactation Database,* National Center for Biotechnology Information, https://www.ncbi.nlm.nih.gov/books/NBK501469/.
6. "Alcohol," *Breastfeeding,* Centers for Disease Control and Prevention, https://www.cdc.gov/breastfeeding/breastfeeding-special-circumstances/vaccinations-medications-drugs/alcohol.html.
7. "Alcohol and Breastfeeding: What's Your Time-to-Zero?," *Breastfeeding,* Infant Risk Center, https://www.infantrisk.com/content/alcohol-breastfeeding-whats-your-time-zero.
8. "Alcohol," *Drugs and Lactation Database* (LactMed®) (Bethesda, MD: National Institute of Child Health and Human Development, 2006– ; updated January 18, 2022), https://www.ncbi.nlm.nih.gov/books/NBK501469/.
9. Rita Patel, Emily Oken, Natalia Bogdanovich, Lidia Matush, Zinaida Sevkovskaya, Beverley Chalmers, Ellen D Hodnett, Konstantin Vilchuck, Michael S Kramer, and Richard M Martin, "Cohort Profile: The Promotion of Breastfeeding Intervention Trial (PROBIT)," *International Journal of Epidemiology* 43, no. 3 (2014): 679–90, https://www.ncbi.nlm.nih.gov/pmc/articles/PMC4052126/.
10. Vanessa Vigar, Stephen Myers, Christopher Oliver, Jacinta Arellano, Shelley Robinson, and Carlo Leifert, "A Systematic Review of Organic Versus Conventional Food Consumption: Is There a Measurable Benefit on Human Health?," *Nutrients* 12, no. 1 (2020): 7, https://www.ncbi.nlm.nih.gov/pmc/articles/PMC7019963/.
11. "Publications of James J. McKenna, PhD," Mother-Baby Behavioral Sleep Laboratory, University of Notre Dame College of Arts and Letters, https://cosleeping.nd.edu/mckenna-biography/list-of-publications/.

12. Helen M. Johnson, Anne Eglash, Katrina B. Mitchell, Kathy Leeper, et al., "ABM Clinical Protocol #32: Management of Hyperlactation," *Breastfeeding Medicine* 15, no. 3 (2020), https://www.liebertpub.com/doi/10.1089/bfm.2019.29141.hmj.
13. Helen M. Johnson, Anne Eglash, Katrina B. Mitchell, Kathy Leeper, et al., "ABM Clinical Protocol #32: Management of Hyperlactation," *Breastfeeding Medicine* 15, no. 3 (2020), https://www.liebertpub.com/doi/10.1089/bfm.2019.29141.hmj.
14. Caroline GA van Veldhuizen-Staas, "Overabundant Milk Supply: An Alternative Way to Intervene by Full Drainage and Block Feeding," *International Breastfeeding Journal* 2 (2007): 11, https://www.ncbi.nlm.nih.gov/pmc/articles/PMC2075483/.
15. Britt Frisk Pados, PhD, RN, NNP-BC, Jinhee Park, PhD, RN, Suzanne M. Thoyre, PhD, RN, FAAN, Hayley Estrem, PhD, RN, and W. Brant Nix, BMET, BA, "Milk Flow Rates from Bottle Nipples Used After Hospital Discharge," *MCN, The American Journal of Maternal/Child Nursing* 41, no. 4 (2016): 237–43, https://www.ncbi.nlm.nih.gov/pmc/articles/PMC5033656/.
16. These techniques come from a combination of the *Journal of Human Lactation* and Francie Webb's book *Go Milk Yourself,* which you should absolutely go read. Genevieve E. Becker and Trudie Roberts, "Do We Agree? Using a Delphi Technique to Develop Consensus on Skills of Hand Expression," *Journal of Human Lactation* 25, no. 2 (2009): 220–225, doi: 10.1177/0890334409333679; Francie Webb, *Go Milk Yourself,* (self-pub., TheMilkinMama, LLC, 2017).
17. Anne Eglash, Liliana Simon, The Academy of Breastfeeding Medicine, et al, "ABM Clinical Protocol #8: Human Milk Storage Information for Home Use for Full-Term Infants, Revised 2017," Breastfeeding Medicine (Sep 2017): 390–95. doi: 10.1089/bfm.2017.29047.aje.
18. Joy Noel-Weiss , A. Kirsten Woodend , Wendy E. Peterson , William Gibb , Dianne L. Groll, "An Observational Study of Associations among Maternal Fluids during Parturition, Neonatal Output, and Breastfed Newborn Weight Loss," *International Breastfeeding Journal* 6, no. 9 (2011), doi: 10.1186/1746-4358-6-9.
19. Markus Heinrichs, Inga Neumann, Ulrike Ehlert, "Lactation and Stress: Protective Effects of Breast-feeding in Humans," *Stress* 5, no. 3 (2002): 195–203. doi: 10.1080/1025389021000010530.
20. J. L. Cox, J. M. Holden, and R. Sagovsky, "Detection of postnatal depression: Development of the 10-item Edinburgh Postnatal Depression Scale," *British Journal of Psychiatry* 150 (1987), 782–786.

INDEX

C

P